HAPPY HEALTHY STRONG

THE SECRET TO STAYING FIT FOR LIFE

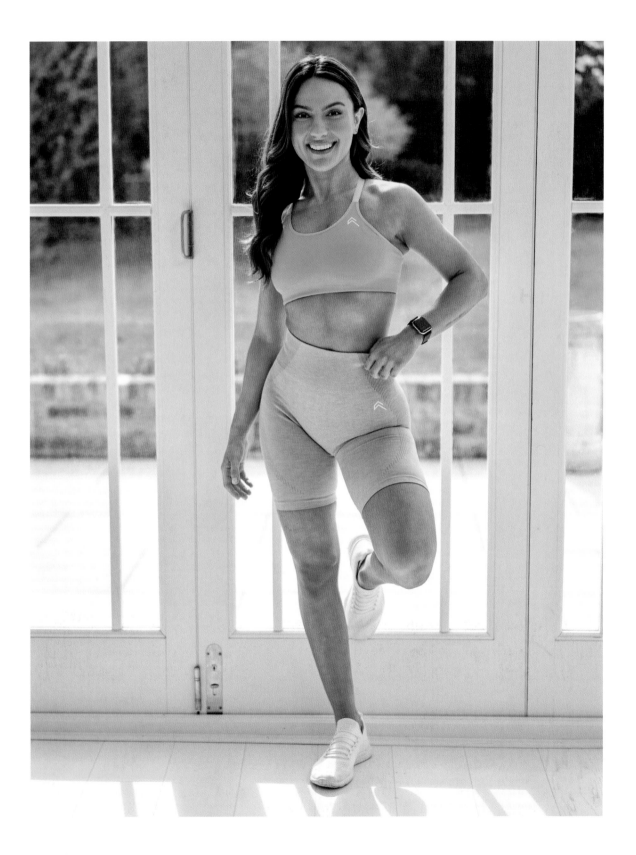

HAPPY HEALTHY STRONG

THE SECRET TO STAYING FIT FOR LIFE

KRISSY CELA

Recipes · Workouts · Expert Advice

Go
hachette
BOOKS
NEW YORK

Copyright © 2021 by Krissy Cela
First published in Great Britain in 2021 by Aster, an imprint of Octopus Publishing Group

Cover design by Octopus Publishing Group
Cover photography by Tamin Jones and Danny Bird

Photographs by Tamin Jones and Danny Bird
Cover copyright © 2021 by Hachette Book Group, Inc.

Hachette Go, an imprint of Hachette Books
Hachette Book Group
1290 Avenue of the Americas
New York, NY 10104
HachetteGo.com
Facebook.com/HachetteGo
Instagram.com/HachetteGo

First Edition: December 2021

Hachette Books is a division of Hachette Book Group, Inc.
The Hachette Go and Hachette Books name and logos are trademarks of Hachette Book Group, Inc.

The publisher is not responsible for websites (or their content) that are not owned by the publisher.

Library of Congress Cataloging-in-Publication Data has been applied for.

ISBNs: 978-0-306-92509-2 (paperback); 978-0-306-92510-8 (ebook)

Library of Congress Control Number: 2021944392

Printed in the United States of America

WOR

10 9 8 7 6 5 4 3 2 1

To my mum, my superhero and
the woman who risked it all…
this is all for you, always will be

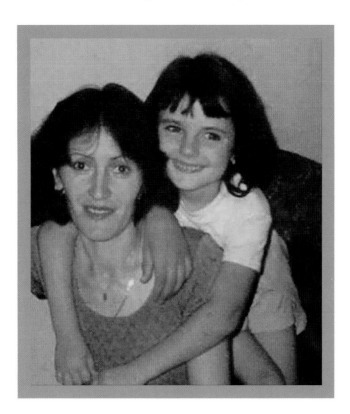

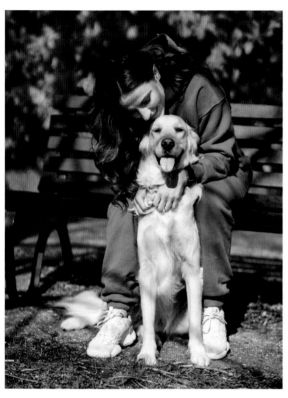
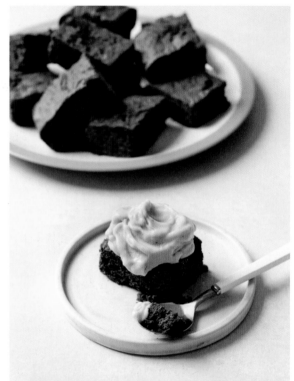
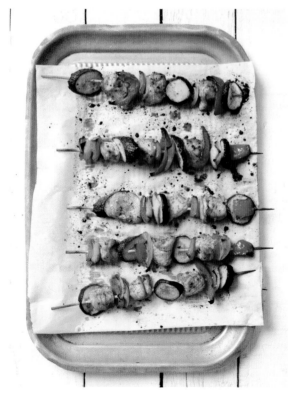
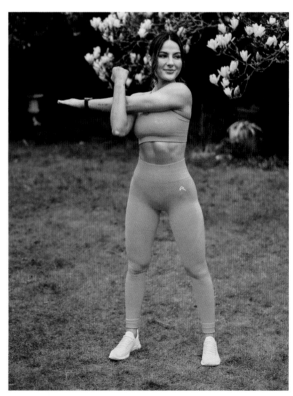

CONTENTS

WELCOME

Hi, familia! Thank you for trusting me to be your trainer. I'm here to teach you that looking after your fitness and health is a sustainable, lifelong choice that can become as natural a part of your routine as brushing your teeth. I can't wait to help you be and love the best version of yourself!

Fitness saved me—I cannot emphasize that enough. When I discovered the gym several years ago and started training, I was blown away by how empowering it can be. I felt strong, I felt healthy, and I felt so happy. For the first time in a long time, I was doing something that was solely for me. No one else mattered—my body, my mind and I came first. When I started tracking my fitness journey online in 2016, I absolutely loved all the women I was meeting and, more than anything, I loved the supportive community we were building. Just like the gym, my online community—my familia—was a space far away from the stress of uni, work and everyday life. I felt strong, confident and happy and, day by day, I wanted to help more and more women feel the same. There is nothing more empowering and satisfying than seeing women work out, build confidence and be the best version of themselves.

I'm determined to help each and every one of you feel happy, healthy and strong—mentally and physically. I'm here for you, and we're all here for each other. I can't wait to see you do this for you!

Krissy Cela

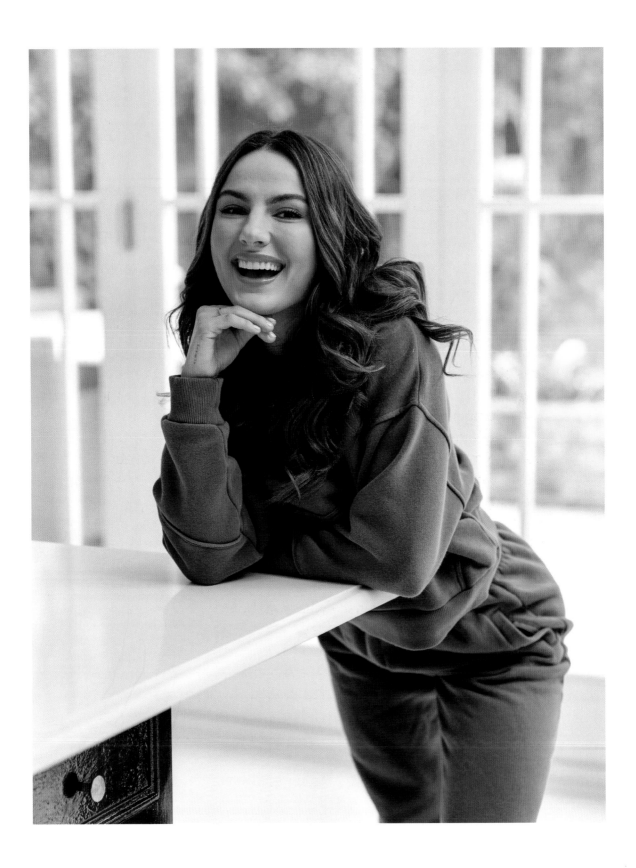

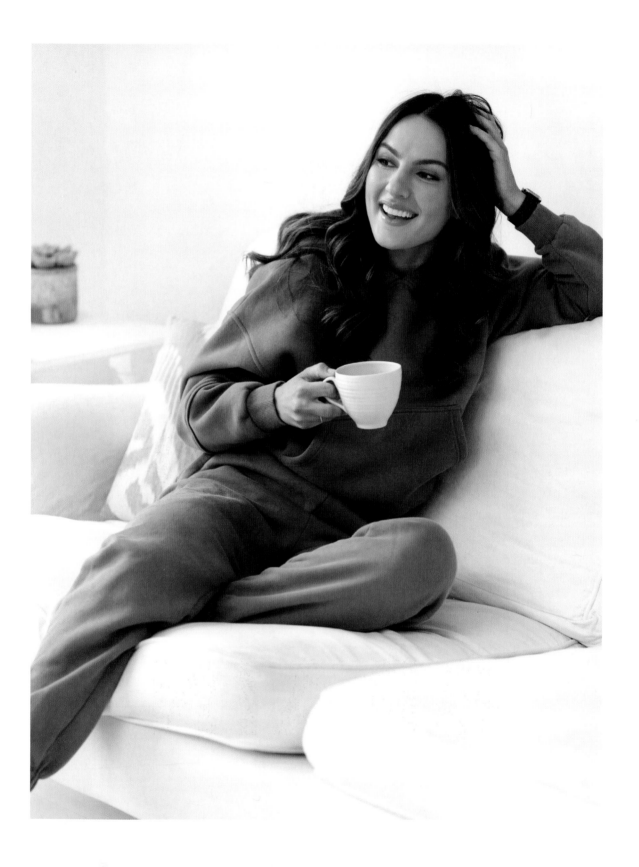

1

TRAIN YOUR BRAIN

PUT YOURSELF FIRST

For too long, women have put themselves last. They have put their happiness last. But little do we know that our happiness really matters. You matter—your health, your well-being, everything about you matters. Sometimes work, the kids, family or friends get in the way of your goals. While these play an important part in your life, *you* play the most important part.

It sounds silly. You're probably thinking, I know I matter, Krissy, that's pretty obvious! But let me ask you this:

- How many times have you rescheduled a gym session to fit in an extra meeting at work?

- How many times have you pushed back your workout because your partner asked you for some help, or the kids needed help with their homework?

- How many times have you chosen to watch television over meal prepping or scheduling your workouts?

Trust me, I see you, I see the penny drop as you realize this is happening more often than it should be! Don't get me wrong, I love watching television and really value time with my friends and family, but spending time with them or getting engrossed in a box set means exactly that: spending time with things and people other than yourself. Think about it: you fit in your job, socials after work, housework, errands, family time…and more work. All of this is functional; it's you getting through life. However, you'll find you burn out, slow down and begin to question what it is you're actually doing on a day-to-day basis.

Before you know it, you're feeling sluggish and frustrated and find yourself questioning your self-worth. You don't feel good enough—in fact, you don't really know what "enough" means anymore. Why? Because you've spent so much time involved in everything around you and not enough time on yourself. You're functioning on autopilot—everything is a process, something that just needs to "get done"—but you don't really know why you're doing it or what you're achieving.

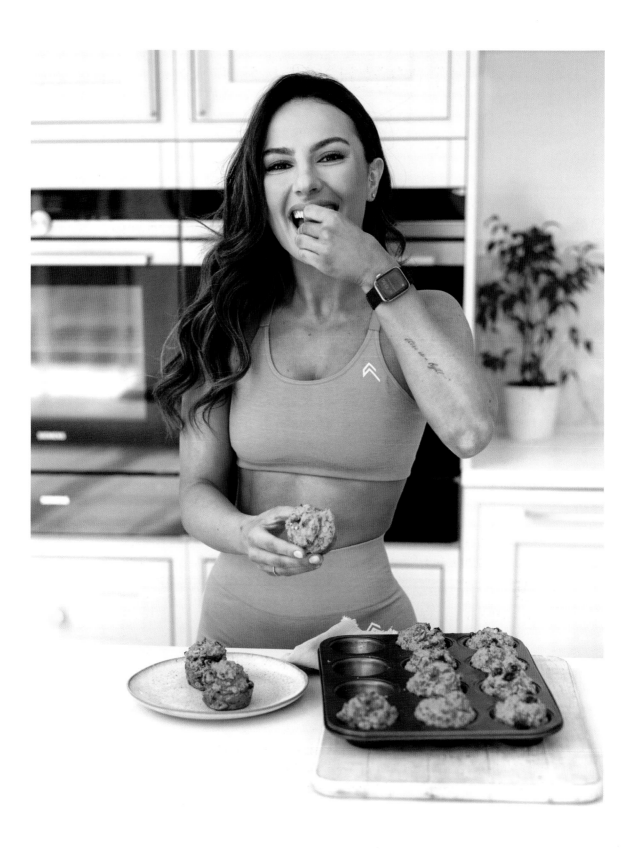

Your Happiness Is Your "Why"

Happiness comes from within you. Happiness is a truly positive and confident state of mind. It's when you feel emotionally, mentally and physically well in yourself. You feel in control. You know what's good for you, and you have the ability to make the best decisions for yourself. So many of us are guilty of people-pleasing or looking for that sense of validation and happiness in other people, other actions and other events. But true happiness starts with you—and what better way to focus on yourself than on your physical and mental well-being?

This book aims to help you understand and learn how to make your happiness a priority by focusing on your fitness. All I want is for you to feel healthy, happy and strong, and I know that is something you can discover and maintain through exercise and a balanced lifestyle. Your fitness journey will become a journey of discovery; you will learn how your body performs, what it enjoys, what it needs, what makes you feel confident, what challenges you, what makes you jump up in the morning and keeps you smiling all day.

I also want you to fall in love with food. Food is fuel, fun and love—food is everything and more for a balanced lifestyle, and it doesn't need to be boring. Let me take you on a journey of flavor, color and wholesome foods, which include protein, fats and carbs—we don't skip a single food group, and we enjoy every one of them! Most importantly, I can't wait to introduce you to Mama Cela's amazing Albanian masterpieces, which can also be a part of a healthy, balanced lifestyle—there is room for it all on your journey to good health.

Longevity over Any Trend

Ask yourself this: Are shredded abs, a sculpted booty or toned triceps the key to happiness? Are they the key to health? The answer is no! The key to your happiness, your "why," is longevity.

• I want you to be running around with your kids and your grandkids in your fifties.

• I want you to be taking the stairs and not the elevator in your sixties.

• I want you to carry your own shopping bag in your seventies.

Fitness is not a trend. Building strong glutes is not for the sake of social media. Having a strong core is not just for summer. Fitness is:

• a healthy heart

• good stamina

• strong bones

• supple joints

• painless movement and mobility

• a healthy mind

Fitness is for life—it is a habit that makes you strong, resilient, confident and able to take on any challenge that life throws at you. It teaches you the patience and discipline necessary to take on the world! It makes you realize you have time for yourself, you have time to be healthy, happy and strong no matter where you are in life.

The workouts, recipes and advice in this book will help you achieve just that: a fit and healthy lifestyle that you can sustain, build and grow. You are worth investing in, so take the time to do this for you. I promise you, you won't regret it.

WHAT IS YOUR "WHY"?

It all starts with a choice—your choice, your decision, your mindset to commit to you. I've said it before, and I'll say it again: exercise is not just about physical strength, it's about mental and emotional strength too. In order to complete any workout, including the workouts in this book, you need to have the mental and emotional stamina to show up, work through it and get it done. People always ask me, "Krissy, I know I'm doing this for me, but how do I keep going? How do I fit it all in? How do I stay motivated? Where do I start?" Well, this chapter will answer all these questions and more!

The first thing I want you to do is remind yourself why you're here. Why are you reading this book? What do you want to achieve? Why do you want fitness to be a happy, healthy and strong lifelong habit? I always say fitness is internal, first, before it can be external: it's about how it makes you feel, what it makes you think and why it makes you the best version of yourself.

However, I totally get it that you might want to look good on vacation, wear your favorite pair of jeans again and love what you see in the mirror. While this is all valid, just remember: internal before external. You will only keep going if it makes you feel great about yourself, and proud. Every rep, every exercise, every movement will get better and better with consistency, and that will become your reason to keep going. Then, the jeans and the vacation just become a part of this holistic and happy lifestyle.

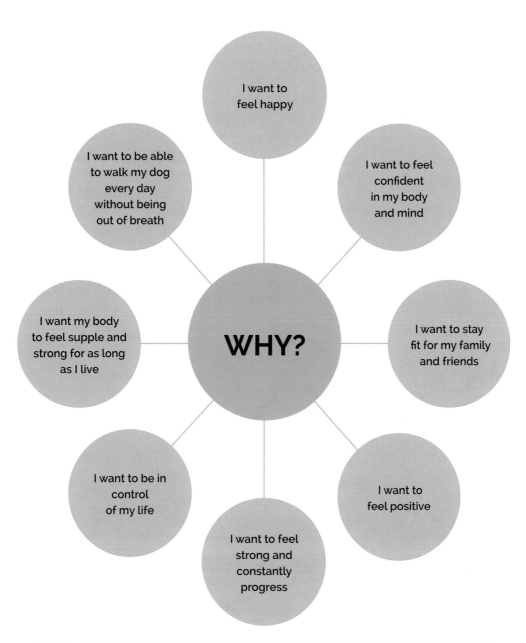

Task: Find your "why"

On a piece of paper, I want you to mind map every reason, everything that makes you want to work out. This is your space to write down anything you like—it will be your reminder of why you've chosen to put yourself first.

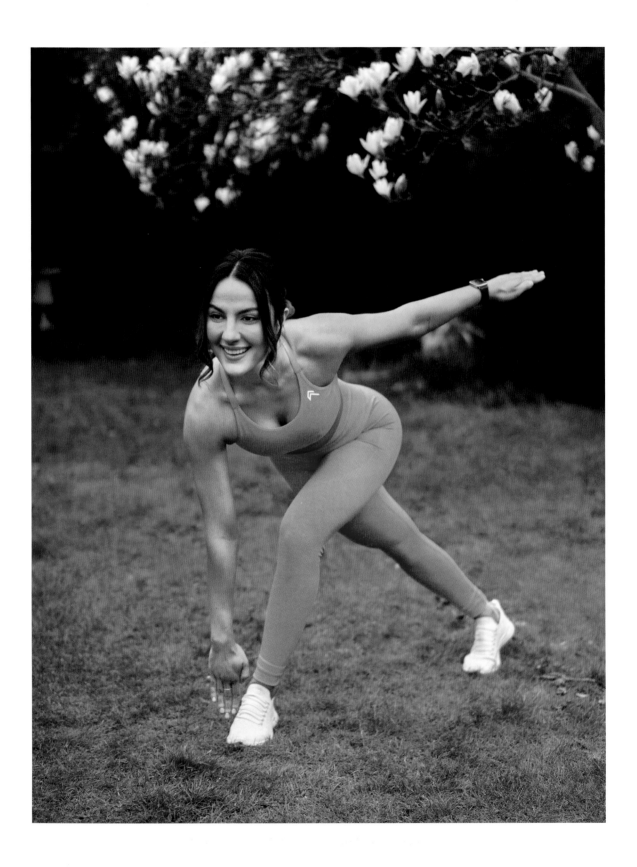

HABITS, SCHEDULING, DISCIPLINE . . . REPEAT

Motivation is short-lived. It comes and goes and is different for everyone. You cannot rely on it to keep you going. How do I stay motivated? I don't, but I keep going anyway. How? Here are my most successful tips.

Healthy Habits

A habit is a second-nature action—it is something you usually form in childhood or when you're growing up and is based on what your parents teach you and on the kind of lifestyle you lead. You need to change up the idea that fitness is an add-on activity and start to believe that it is a habit for life. Remember your mum always telling you to eat breakfast before you leave the house or to stop biting your nails? Well, just as those things have become lifelong habits for you, I want you to develop a habit of fitting in your workout every day.

Habits never let you down—you do them without thinking, and you love them because they make you who you are. Without your habits, you feel incomplete—that's exactly how I want you to see exercise. So, how do you form a healthy habit? Practice!

If fitness is brand-new for you, I want you to start by committing just fifteen minutes a day to exercise. You could go for a run or a walk, or complete some of the exercises in the Move Move Move section later in the book (see page 183). You need to do fifteen minutes of exercise every day for at least a month. Contrary to popular belief, a habit doesn't take a fixed amount of time to form—some say it takes three weeks, some say twelve weeks, some say six weeks—so just keep doing the fifteen minutes a day for as long as you need until the habit becomes ingrained. You will start to notice a difference in mind and body. I want you to look forward to those fifteen minutes, to work on yourself and be the very best version of you.

At the beginning, commit to doing the same exercise every day for at least seven days. For example, you might choose to run every day for the first week, complete strength exercises every day during the second week, then go back to running in the third week, and do more strength exercises in the fourth week.

The Importance of Repetition

The reasons I'm advising you to repeat the exercises are:

- **Habits need to be second nature**—the less you have to think about them, the more likely you are to get up and do them.

- **Consistency is the key to success**—the more you stick to an exercise, the more you will notice progress in your mental and physical strength.

- **It takes time to figure out what you enjoy**. We are so used to instant gratification, but exercise takes time to fall in love with—all the best things do!

Scheduling

When forming a healthy habit, your routine is of the utmost importance. Once you take control of your schedule and your time, you won't need to worry about motivation or how to fit it all in.

Grab a monthly, weekly and daily planner with squares big enough for you to write in. If possible, choose one with hour slots throughout the day. Fill in your planner with everything you have to do on a weekly basis. Be specific and put in times too. For example, if you have a college day, write in the times of your classes; if you are going to work, don't forget to list your commute time.

Now schedule in two sessions in the week for your food prep, one on a Sunday and one midweek. Find two slots of about two hours each, in which you can decide what you're going to eat that week and spend time preparing ahead and batch cooking. Check out the Fuel Your Life section (see page 29) for inspiration. Now find the time in your schedule every day to do at least fifteen minutes or more of exercise and write it in. I recommend every day so you can make exercise a habit, and I say "or more" because there will be some days when you will have time to commit to doing a little more than fifteen minutes. There may also be some days when you do less, and that is OK too as long as you are getting something in every day—movement is key. Take a look at my schedule to give you an idea.

Day/Time	Monday	Tuesday	Wednesday	Thursday	Friday	Saturday	Sunday
6:30am	Wake up & walk the dog	Wake up & walk the dog	Wake up & walk the dog	Wake up & walk the dog	Wake up & walk the dog	Sleep in	Sleep in
7am	Get ready & breakfast	Get ready & breakfast	Get ready & breakfast	Get ready & breakfast	Get ready & breakfast		
8am	Travel to work	Work	Travel to work	Travel to work	Recording video content	Get ready & breakfast	Get ready & breakfast
9am	Work		Work	Work		Walk the dog	Walk the dog
10am	Work	Recording video content	Work	Work		Work out	Schedule next week
11am							
12pm							
1pm	Lunch	Lunch	Lunch	Lunch	Lunch	Lunch	Lunch
2pm	Meetings	Recording video content	Meetings	Meetings	Recording video content		Meal prep
3pm							
4pm							
5pm	Travel home	Meal prep	Travel home	Travel home			
6pm	Work out		Walk the dog	Work out	Dinner with Hollie		
7pm	Dinner	Dinner	Work out	Dinner			
8pm	Walk the dog	Walk the dog	Dinner	Walk the dog	Walk the dog	Dinner	Dinner
9pm	Chill & unwind before bed	Chill & unwind before bed	Chill & unwind before bed	Chill & unwind before bed	Chill & unwind before bed		
10pm							
11:30pm	Shower & bed	Shower & bed	Shower & bed	Shower & bed	Shower & bed	Shower & bed	Shower & bed

Now that you've seen an example of my schedule, think about your own schedule and consider the following:

- Where could you fit in your workouts?

- When could you meal prep?

- When could you plan for the weeks and days ahead?

Looking at your whole week together can really help you put an effective routine in place. I walk Buttons every day, which means I definitely get fifteen minutes or more of movement in. I like to strength-train three or four times a week, so I look at my schedule and work out where I can fit in those sessions. Here are a few things to consider when scheduling your workouts:

- **When do you like to train?** Some people say it's better to train in the morning, but my body clock tells me I prefer training in the evening.

- **How long are you going to train?** I've asked you to put in fifteen minutes, because everyone can find fifteen minutes in their day. However, even for me, there are some days where I'm going to be tight on time. Don't worry! Tailor your workout to suit you—it's the only way you'll stay consistent.

- **What do you want to train?** Planning your workouts is key. I cannot emphasize that enough. Your workout will be one thousand times more effective if you turn up to it with a plan. You'll finish your workout knowing you've trained the areas you want to target and you'll feel so much better for it. See pages 184–190 for tips on planning your workout.

Finally, the other thing I factor in my schedule is time set aside for planning the following week. This is super important to keep me consistent and successful, so always make time to plan ahead and write it in your schedule.

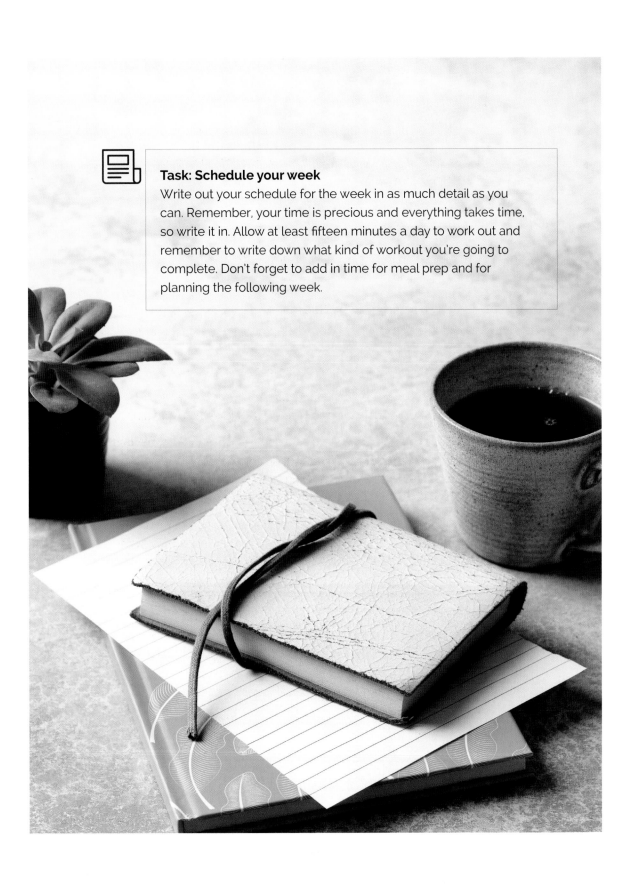

Task: Schedule your week

Write out your schedule for the week in as much detail as you can. Remember, your time is precious and everything takes time, so write it in. Allow at least fifteen minutes a day to work out and remember to write down what kind of workout you're going to complete. Don't forget to add in time for meal prep and for planning the following week.

Discipline

With your schedule now complete, all you need is discipline to stick to your routine. Healthy habits and a schedule to suit you will immediately make you feel happier. You will feel you have control over your time, your mind and your body. You have fit in things to suit you and your lifestyle. It's quite possibly the most liberating thing you can do for yourself on a daily basis. I know that sounds a little over the top, but it's true! Soon enough, your schedule will become your routine. For example:

- If you schedule your workouts at roughly the same time every day, you're more likely to stick to them, and you'll know that that time is your time.

- When other people ask for your time or if a friend asks to schedule a coffee, instead of saying yes to anything and everything, you're more likely to take control of your time and do things on your terms. This isn't selfish, it's self-care!

- You'll know more about yourself. Your routine means you'll know when to say yes and when to say no. The most frustrating and anxious feeling is rushing from task to task, person to person, not being able to catch your breath. It's important to take control for your mental and emotional health.

- Your routine will be consistent, so your sleep cycle will be better, your eating habits will be healthier and you'll just feel happier.

However, for any of this to work, you need discipline. We all have those days when no matter how organized our schedules are, all we want to do is chuck it out the window and stay in bed; no matter how well planned our workouts are, all we want to do is relax on the sofa and eat chocolate. I have those days too. You know what I do? I follow my schedule anyway. It's hard, yes, but you'll never regret that workout. You'll remind yourself of just how strong you are and how much you can accomplish. Plus, the chocolate and duvet will still be there when you've finished. Just stay consistent, stay strong and get it done—you'll feel so much better afterward.

PLANNING &
PROBLEM-SOLVING

The key to a happy lifestyle is planning. Writing lists can be therapeutic. It's a way of taking control—you then decide how, why and when you're going to tackle your list. Making lists can help you plan and prioritize your well-being. Honestly, you will love how much more peaceful you feel.

Task: List your problems

Every night, write down everything that is playing on your mind—all the tasks you have to do, any problems and even happy things. Give yourself five to ten minutes to write everything out.

In the morning, look at the list again. Now, with a refreshed mind, I want you to plan how you are going to tackle five of the items on your list. You can add them to your schedule if necessary.

Problem	Solution	Action Plan
I haven't worked out in three days, and I'm feeling really sluggish. I have no idea when or how to fit a workout in. Life is so busy.	I won't beat myself up about it. Life happens and it can be fixed. I could: • Wake up 30 minutes earlier to fit a workout in • Do a 15-minute workout at lunchtime • Go for a run after work	I will add workouts to next week's schedule when I'm planning my week.

SMALL STEPS TO HAPPINESS

We often let big dreams get in the way of our happiness. Let me give you some examples. We spend so much time thinking, "I want to get fit to run a marathon," that we let the marathon take over our lives. Or we might think, "The only way to train is by lifting really heavy weights," and all we focus on is our personal best.

As much as these thoughts and goals are valid, we let them get in the way of our everyday, small wins—and that isn't what fitness should be.

Approaching fitness with a holistic mind is all about small changes, small steps, all designed to make you feel and be your very best. That might be eating more veggies every day, making your own lunch instead of buying it or taking the stairs instead of the elevator. These steps are the key to feeling positive and happy about fitness—not putting pressure on yourself when you're working out.

Task: Take stock
I want you to take a few minutes every day to think about the things you've done to contribute to your fitness journey. It might be a fifteen-minute workout or a thirty-minute run; it might be a workout from this book; it might be walking to work instead of taking the bus. Whatever it is, give yourself a few minutes every day to remind yourself that you are doing the very best for you— that is true happiness!

So What's the Key to Happiness?

You. You are your best friend, your best cheerleader, your best you! Prioritizing your fitness journey, your food and your health will help everything else fall into place. You'll feel more confident in yourself; you'll take control of your own time, decisions and choices. We all spend so much time focusing on the happiness of others, but now I want you to make your life, your well-being, the number one priority. And the beauty of it is, it doesn't take very long! People think you need to train for hours on end in the gym, but a simple thirty- to forty-minute workout at home or at the gym is all you need to get those endorphins going to make you feel great about yourself. If you start with fifteen minutes, you'll soon realize you have time to fit in another fifteen minutes. Just start making time for your well-being and, I promise you, those happy feelings will follow.

You just need to focus on:

- your "whys"

- your habits

- your schedule

- your routine

- your planning

Remember to grab a diary, a journal or the calendar on your phone and schedule your workouts. When it's set in stone (in black and white), you're way more likely to do the workout as the planning and thinking have already been done. And if you're not feeling it? Just get up and do it anyway—remember, it's a healthy habit, one that you will never regret.

Get your mindset right using my tips, and your workouts and meal planning will soon feel as natural as brushing your teeth. I can't wait to see the positive changes you make to your lifestyle, and I am here with you every step of the way.

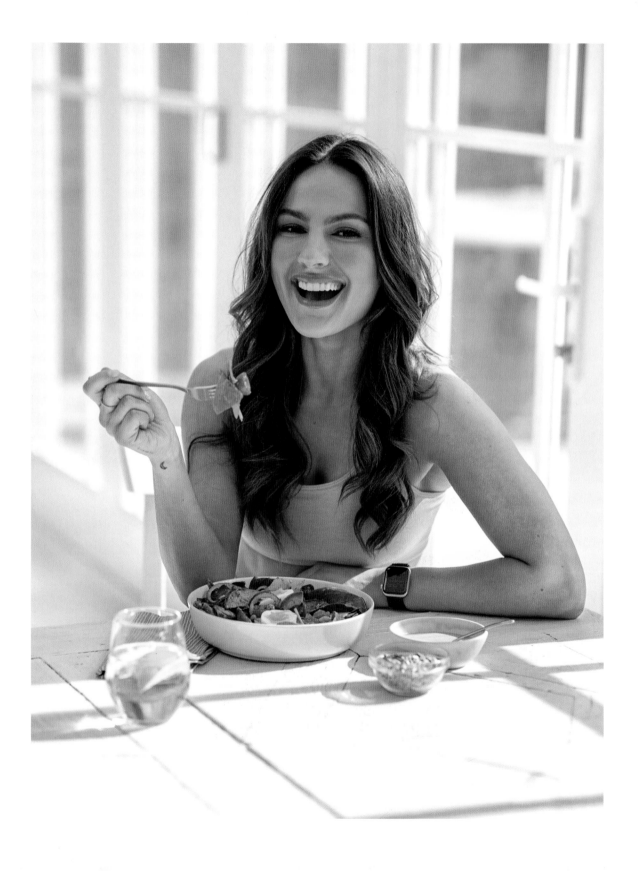

2

FUEL
YOUR
LIFE

THE IMPORTANCE OF FOOD

Food fuels your body, but what about cooking? Cooking is food for your soul! There is nothing I enjoy more than putting on my favorite playlist, dancing around the kitchen, and cooking up a nutritious and mouth-watering meal. When I was younger, mealtimes were a real celebration. We didn't inhale our food while our minds were elsewhere; we enjoyed every single flavorsome bite my mum put on our plates—it's what I miss most about living at home with my parents.

I often hear women talking about going on a diet, cutting out carbs, eating celery and tiny portions or feeling hungry, miserable and lethargic because they're trying to "lose weight."

But it's simple: food = energy. We need energy to:

- work

- sleep

- talk to friends

- take care of the kids

- keep our brains active and engaged

- exercise

- be stress-free

- be happy

So we need to eat—food is not something we should deprive ourselves of. Instead, we need to learn about it and understand why good nutrition is so important for us.

WHAT DOES IT MEAN TO BE HEALTHY?

Let's take a minute to look at the word "healthy." Personally, for a long time I had a problem with the word. Why? Because I felt like there was only one version of healthy, and I wasn't it. We now live in a world where the media and supermarkets tell us what healthy is—and we believe it. It's almost like there is no room to have balance or create a lifestyle that works for your health.

Education about food is key. You need to know why you're fueling your body, what amazing things food does for you, and why it's OK to enjoy your favorite treats while eating a wholesome and balanced diet.

The purpose of this book and my recipes is to do just that—help you find the balance and learn to eat intuitively. By that, I mean to eat when you are hungry, but eat a balanced meal so you feel satiated. And one bar of chocolate or a donut doesn't ruin everything! Of course, if you have specific health concerns that affect your nutrition, you should consult a doctor.

Everything in moderation. Having discipline when it comes to food is key. The choices you make need to be balanced. It's OK to pop some chocolate in your cart during your food shop, but make sure you also visit the fresh fruit and veggie aisle and stock up on those too. Balance is key!

Just remember to enjoy your food, define your own version of healthy, and find a balance that works for your health and happiness.

WHAT IS GOOD & BAD NUTRITION?

There isn't really such a thing as good and bad nutrition—the word "bad" shouldn't be used when it comes to food, as it leads to a toxic relationship with food, which can cause yo-yo dieting and your health becoming a short-term fix as opposed to a lifelong journey. Food shouldn't be something you're scared of. The amount of times I see women hesitate over portion sizes, a chocolate bar or a pizza—I just want to give them a big hug and teach them food is not the enemy. When you learn about the different food groups, what your body needs and what will keep you feeling energized, you'll know what's good for you and what healthy means to you.

Nutritional Value

The words "good" and "bad" have been used to define different nutritional values. Different foods obviously contain different levels of a range of nutrients and, over time, this has led so many to say pizza is bad for you and broccoli is good for you. It's not as simple as that. Yes, broccoli is a good source of fiber, contains some protein, and can provide many of the vitamins and micronutrients our bodies need, but eating a ton of broccoli won't make you healthy overnight. Similarly, avocados are a good source of monounsaturated fatty acids (great for heart health, nutrient absorption and reducing inflammation), but eating lots of them does not mean you're eating a balanced diet. Likewise, there is a difference between eating a couple slices of pizza and eating a whole pizza—that's not balanced either!

So no foods are all "good" or all "bad"—all of them can play a part in our diets, as long as we strike a healthy balance. Processed foods are the ones we want to be more mindful of. Yes we can eat them, but nutritionally dense foods—the foods we need to fuel our workouts and keep us energized and full for longer—will come from a more balanced plate.

What Are Processed Foods?

In a nutshell, processed foods are ones that come ready made, ready to serve. Think deep-fried foods, burgers, fries, pizzas, ready-made pasta sauces, frozen meals, chocolate and potato chips.

Remember, I'm not saying these foods are "bad," I'm saying they are not nutritionally dense enough to eat on a regular basis. They don't contain the macronutrients, vitamins and minerals we need, and they can leave us feeling tired, bloated and dehydrated. Plus, unless we study every ingredients list, we don't always know what we're putting into our bodies. I like to know what I'm eating!

We need to approach our food and our recipes with our health and balance in mind. Look at each plate, each snack, and consider its nutritional value—we want our food to leave us feeling energized, satiated and satisfied. We want the nutritional content to be varied with a combination of macro- and micronutrients (see page 37). And we want it to taste delicious too! In a nutshell, we want food to give us energy and fuel our bodies, not zap our energy and make us feel tired or bloated.

Protein

Protein helps to build muscle and it also helps to keep us feeling full, so we should eat protein with every meal. Examples of good sources of protein include red meat, white meat, fish, lentils, beans, eggs, nuts and seeds.

Fats

Fats are high in energy and help our bodies absorb necessary vitamins and minerals. We need fat in our diets to provide certain essential fatty acids. Fat is not the enemy, but as it provides lots of energy, we don't need very much of it—just a thumb-sized portion at each meal. Think a nice drizzle of olive oil, half an avocado or a handful of seeds and nuts. We need to be mindful of fatty foods such as full-fat cream, cakes, cookies, pies, chocolate or too many pizzas! This is because these foods contain trans and saturated fats and can increase the risk of heart disease and other illnesses.

Carbohydrates

Carbohydrates provide energy for our cells. Carbohydrates come in three forms: starch, fiber and sugar.

- **Starchy foods** Think bread, potatoes, pasta, whole-grain foods—what some people call "beige foods"! Whole-grain varieties (brown bread, brown rice, whole wheat pasta) tend to be preferable as they are less processed and are good sources of fiber, which is good for our health and energy levels. Starchy foods, particularly whole-grain varieties, release energy slowly, keeping us fuller for longer—that's why we should not cut out carbs!

- **Fiber** The carbs we eat, especially whole-grain carbs, contain fiber. Fiber is great for our digestion and can help prevent certain health problems, such as type 2 diabetes and heart disease. It also helps us feel fuller for longer. Think whole grains at breakfast and lunch—like oatmeal and brown rice— and loads of veggies at dinner, like broccoli, eggplant, zucchini, peppers and leafy greens. Always eat a rainbow.

- **Sugar** This is the most controversial type of carb! Let me start by saying there are naturally occurring sugars in most of the foods we eat. From fruit to pasta, there is sugar in all of them. This does not make these foods "bad"; it's just another type of energy our bodies need to process. However, we do need to be mindful of added sugars. Think fruit juice, chocolate, cake, syrups and pasta sauces (many processed foods contain added sugar). Added sugar can cause an imbalance on our plates—what we want is to lead a balanced and healthy lifestyle with a good amount of protein, carbs and fats.

However…

This is a general guide and nutritional needs differ from person to person. If we are trying to lose fat and gain muscle, we might increase the amount of protein on our plate and reduce the amount of carbs. If we are trying to increase the level of fiber in our diet, we will eat more veggies and fruit throughout the day. The most important lesson here is to understand what we're eating and why we're eating it; know what we're fueling our bodies with; learn about how different foods can support our well-being; and, most of all, enjoy and love the food we eat. OK, maybe that's more than one lesson!

I am so excited to share some of my favorite recipes with you. I have created each recipe with you in mind—I want you to try new flavors, enjoy the process, and realize that your own home-cooked food can be wholesome, balanced and everything you need. You'll also find a couple of my mum's most amazing meals in here, and I hope you love them just as much as I do!

Understanding the Recipes in This Book

To help you eat a wholesome and balanced diet, each of the recipes in this book contains a nutritional information box. This box tells you the quantity of calories, carbohydrates, fat and protein in each dish. These quantities represent one serving of each recipe and include all parts of the recipe such as marinades and dressing. They do not include optional ingredients or serving suggestions.

Planning Ahead and Batch Cooking

As you'll know from having read the first chapter in this book, I am always planning ahead! The same applies to my food and cooking. I like to plan what I'm eating each week. Whenever possible, I make my meals in batches and keep them in the refrigerator or freezer—ready for those busy days when I don't have time to cook. That way, I know I am always getting a nutritious and balanced diet, however hectic my week gets. Many of the recipes in this book can be increased in size to provide more servings, so do bear this in mind when you're creating your own weekly meal plans.

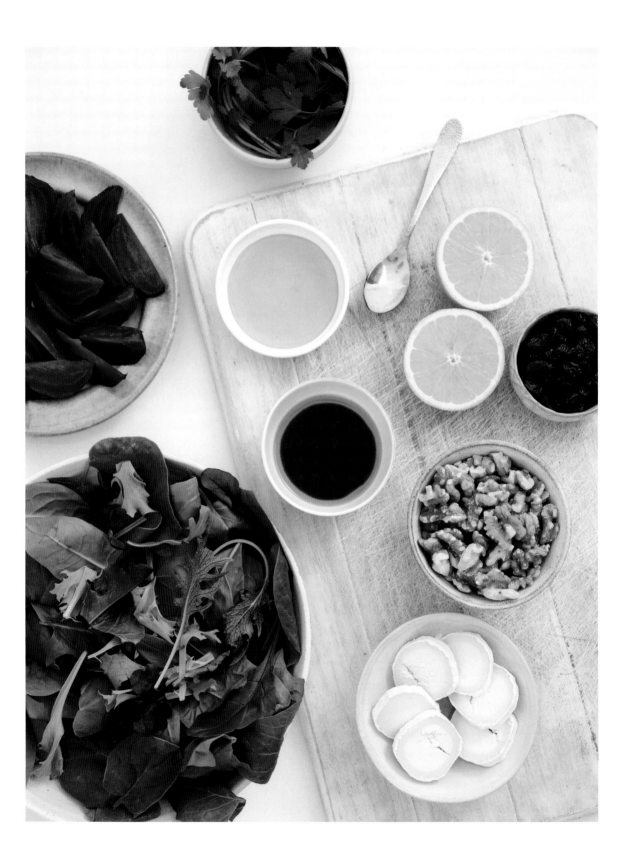

What Is a Balanced Plate?

A balanced plate comprises protein, fats and carbohydrates (known as macronutrients); and vitamins and minerals (known as micronutrients). Micronutrients are found in macronutrients.

Put simply, in order to eat well and sustain healthy eating patterns, we want to ensure our meals are made up of

- a palm-sized portion of protein to build and maintain muscles;

- a cupped hand-sized portion of carbohydrates to provide energy for our cells;

- a thumb-sized portion of fat to help absorb key vitamins and minerals; and

- two handfuls of green veggies to provide loads of key vitamins, minerals and fiber.

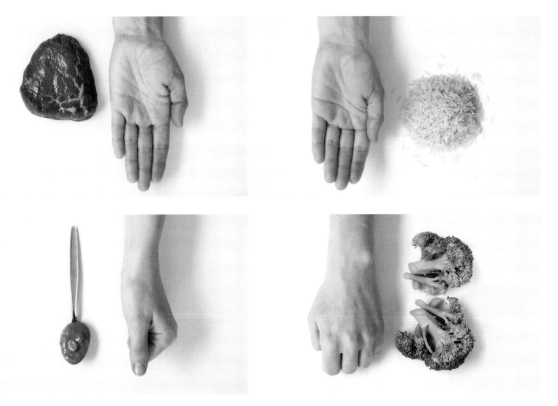

BREAKFAST & BRUNCH

NO-BAKE GRANOLA BREAKFAST BARS

makes 12 bars

10 mins, plus freezing   **5 mins**

These breakfast bars are so simple and easy to make. I love making a batch so that if I'm in a rush, I can just grab one and enjoy breakfast on my way out. Filled with all your key nutrients, along with some sweetness, you'll be snacking on these after breakfast too.

Calories: 462 kcal · Carbohydrates: 45 g · Fat: 28 g · Protein: 10.9 g

5 tablespoons coconut oil
2 tablespoons peanut butter
⅔ cup honey or maple syrup
2 teaspoons vanilla extract
pinch of salt
4½ cups rolled oats
2½ cups toasted coconut flakes

1 cup almonds or other nuts, chopped
¾ cup seeds, such as pumpkin, sunflower or hemp
½ cup dried apricots or cranberries
⅓ cup dark chocolate, chopped

1. Line a 9-inch baking pan with parchment paper.

2. Put the coconut oil, peanut butter, honey or maple syrup, vanilla extract and salt in a saucepan and heat gently for about 2 minutes until the coconut oil has melted. Stir well and remove from the heat.

3. Add the rest of the ingredients and stir until everything is thoroughly coated. Transfer the mixture to the prepared pan and spread evenly with a spatula or the back of a spoon, pressing down until smooth.

4. Place in the freezer for 30 minutes, then remove from the pan and cut into 12 bars.

5. Keep the bars in an airtight container in the freezer for up to 3 weeks. Take one out about 20 minutes before you want to eat it. Alternatively, store at room temperature for up to 7 days.

☑ TIP
Cover the bars in melted dark chocolate.

CARROT CAKE MUFFINS

¶¶ makes 12 muffins

10 mins   **25 mins**

These muffins are absolutely delicious and super easy to make. It's like having dessert for breakfast, and I can't tell you how much I love dessert! Just be sure not to finish the whole batch in one go.

Calories: 301 kcal · Carbohydrates: 31 g · Fat: 17.9 g · Protein: 5.9 g

½ cup olive oil or melted coconut oil, plus extra for greasing
3½ cups rolled oats
⅓ cup pitted dates
4 tablespoons honey or maple syrup

3 large carrots, scrubbed and grated
2 eggs
1 teaspoon baking powder
1 teaspoon ground cinnamon
½ teaspoon grated nutmeg

pinch of salt
¾ cup almond milk, or other milk of your choice
1 cup chopped walnuts
¾ cup raisins

1. Preheat the oven to 350°F (180°C), grease a 12-hole muffin pan.

2. Put all the ingredients, except the walnuts and raisins, in a blender or food processor and blend to form a coarse batter that still has some chunks. Stir in the walnuts and raisins.

3. Divide the mixture between the holes in the muffin pan. Bake for 25 minutes or until the muffins bounce back when you lightly press the tops. Transfer to a wire rack to cool.

4. Store in an airtight container for up to 7 days.

✍ TIP

Make a simple cream cheese icing to spread on the muffins by mixing the finely grated zest and juice of 1 lemon with 2 tablespoons of cream cheese and 1 teaspoon of maple syrup.

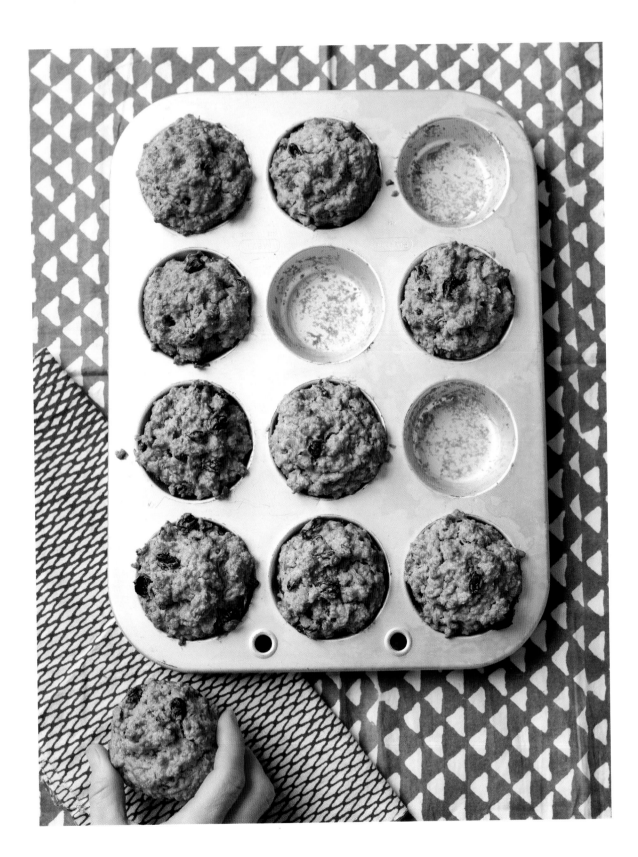

SMOOTHIES

I love a smoothie. These are packed with nutrients and will kick-start your mornings with so much flavor! Feel free to add a scoop of your favorite vanilla protein powder to any of these smoothies. If you like your smoothies very thick, leave out the water.

SALTED CARAMEL SMOOTHIE

🍴 makes 1 large smoothie
👨‍🍳 10 mins

Calories: 362 kcal · Carbohydrates: 64.4 g · Fat: 11.1 g · Protein: 6.9 g

1 cup almond milk, or other milk of your choice

⅔ cup water

1 ripe banana

3–4 pitted dates

1 tablespoon peanut butter

1 teaspoon ground cinnamon

1 teaspoon vanilla extract

large pinch of salt

6 ice cubes

1. Place all the ingredients in a blender or food processor and blend until smooth.

GREEN GODDESS SMOOTHIE

🍴 makes 1 large smoothie
👨‍🍳 10 mins

Calories: 561 kcal · Carbohydrates: 67.8 g · Fat: 33.9 g · Protein: 9.8 g

1 cup almond milk, or other milk of your choice

⅔ cup water

1 small ripe avocado

1 small ripe banana

1 apple, cored and chopped

50 g spinach leaves

1 tablespoon chia seeds

50 g almonds

1 teaspoon spirulina or super greens powder

1 teaspoon vanilla extract

½ teaspoon ground cinnamon

6 ice cubes

1. Place all the ingredients in a blender or food processor and blend until smooth.

MANGO & VANILLA SMOOTHIE

makes 1 large smoothie

10 mins

Calories: 424 kcal · Carbohydrates: 93 g · Fat: 8.2 g · Protein: 4.1 g

1 cup coconut milk, or other milk of your choice

⅔ cup water

1 small ripe banana

2 pitted dates

1¾ cups frozen mango

1 tablespoon chia seeds

1 teaspoon vanilla extract

1 teaspoon ground cinnamon

pinch of salt

½ teaspoon ground turmeric

6 ice cubes

1. Place all the ingredients in a blender or food processor and blend until smooth.

ICED LATTE SMOOTHIE

makes 1 large smoothie

10 mins

Calories: 550 kcal · Carbohydrates: 104.1 g · Fat: 16.9 g · Protein: 8.3 g

1 cup almond milk, or other milk of your choice

1 small ripe banana

4 pitted dates

1 tablespoon chia seeds

1 tablespoon peanut or almond butter

1 teaspoon vanilla extract

1 shot of espresso

6 ice cubes

1. Place all the ingredients in a blender or food processor and blend until smooth.

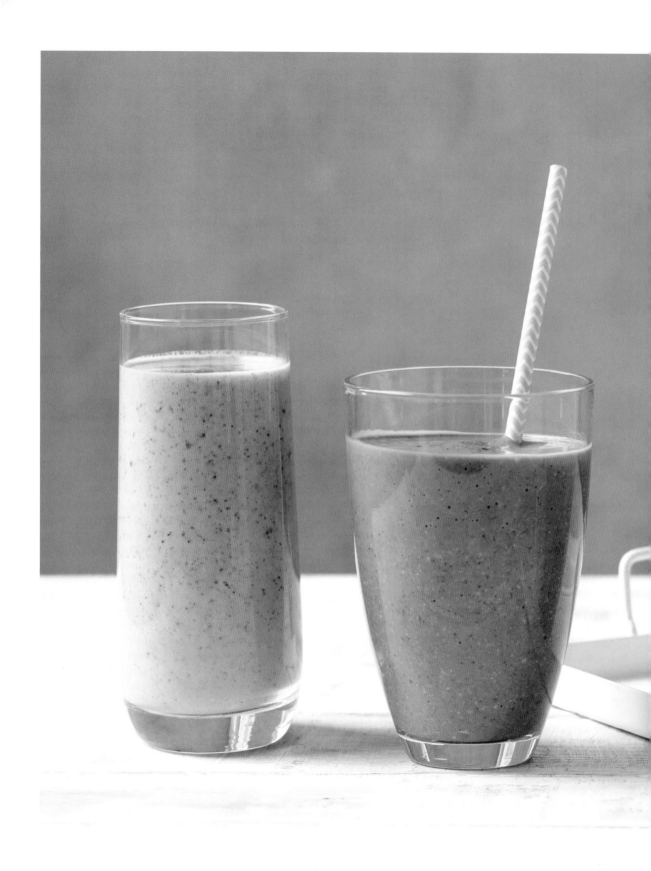

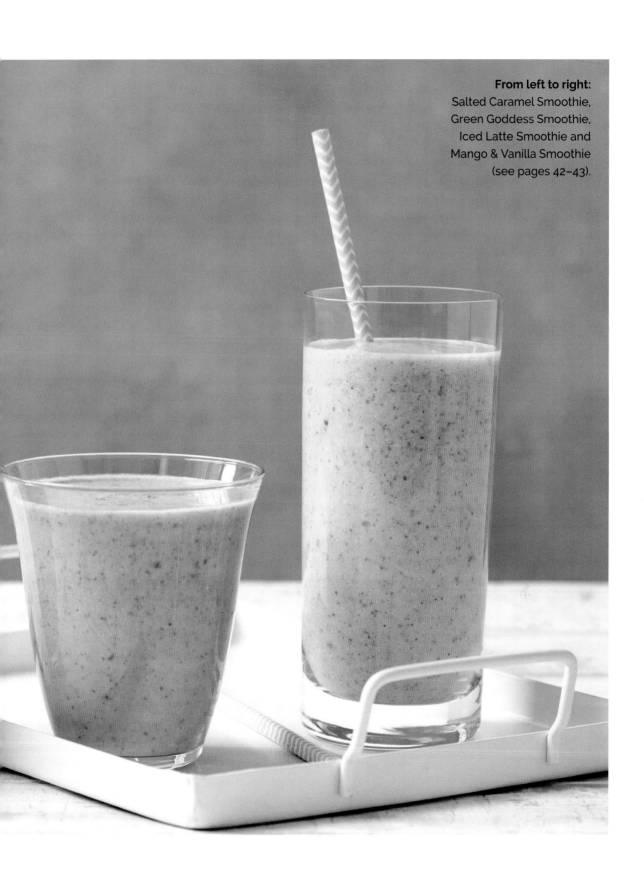

From left to right:
Salted Caramel Smoothie,
Green Goddess Smoothie,
Iced Latte Smoothie and
Mango & Vanilla Smoothie
(see pages 42–43).

OVERNIGHT OATS

🍴 serves 1
👨‍🍳 10 mins, plus chilling

This is my go-to breakfast almost every day. Oats are so nourishing, and with just a few yummy extras they taste delicious. Throw this together the night before and you'll be dreaming about your oats all night long. Banoffee pie is my favorite—of course I'm going to create a breakfast with PIE in it!

Calories: 249 kcal · Carbohydrates: 38 g · Fat: 6.6 g · Protein: 12 g

½ cup rolled oats
⅔ cup plant-based milk of your choice
   (I like coconut milk)
1 teaspoon chia seeds
1 teaspoon ground cinnamon
1 teaspoon vanilla extract
1 teaspoon honey or maple syrup

1. Mix the oats, milk, chia seeds, cinnamon and vanilla in a small jar or bowl and stir in the honey or maple syrup. Cover and chill in the refrigerator overnight. The next morning, add your choice of topping.

STRAWBERRY CHEESECAKE OVERNIGHT OATS

🍴 serves 1
👨‍🍳 5 mins

♡ Overnight Oats plus topping
Calories: 548 kcal · Carbohydrates: 63.3 g · Fat: 23.3 g · Protein: 19.2 g

¾ cup strawberries, chopped
⅔ cup Greek yogurt
1 quantity of Overnight Oats (see above)
1 digestive or oat cookie (I use
   a ginger oat cookie), crushed

1. Mix half the strawberries with the yogurt and stir into the overnight oats. In a jar or bowl, layer the crushed cookie, oats and remaining strawberries and enjoy.

BANOFFEE PIE OVERNIGHT OATS

🍴 serves **1**

👨‍🍳 **10 mins**

♡ Overnight Oats plus topping

Calories: 468 kcal · Carbohydrates: 65.7 g · Fat: 15.7 g · Protein: 15 g

Caramel:
2 pitted dates, soaked in hot water for 5 minutes
½ teaspoon maple syrup
¼ cup almond milk, or other milk of your choice
1 heaped teaspoon peanut or almond butter
pinch of salt (optional)

1 quantity of Overnight Oats (see opposite)
1 small banana, sliced
1 square (about 10 g) of dark chocolate

1. To make the caramel, drain the dates, place in a blender or food processor with the other caramel ingredients and blend until smooth.

2. In a jar or bowl, layer the overnight oats, banana and caramel. Grate the dark chocolate over the top and enjoy.

BLUEBERRY OVERNIGHT OATS

🍴 serves **1**

👨‍🍳 **5 mins**

♡ Overnight Oats plus topping

Calories: 524 kcal · Carbohydrates: 59.5 g · Fat: 22.8 g · Protein: 20.6 g

¾ cup blueberries
⅔ cup Greek yogurt
1 quantity of Overnight Oats (see opposite)
drizzle of honey
1 teaspoon chopped nuts

1. Mix half the blueberries with the yogurt, using a fork to crush the berries so the yogurt turns purple. In a jar or bowl, layer the overnight oats with the blueberry yogurt and remaining blueberries. Top with honey and nuts.

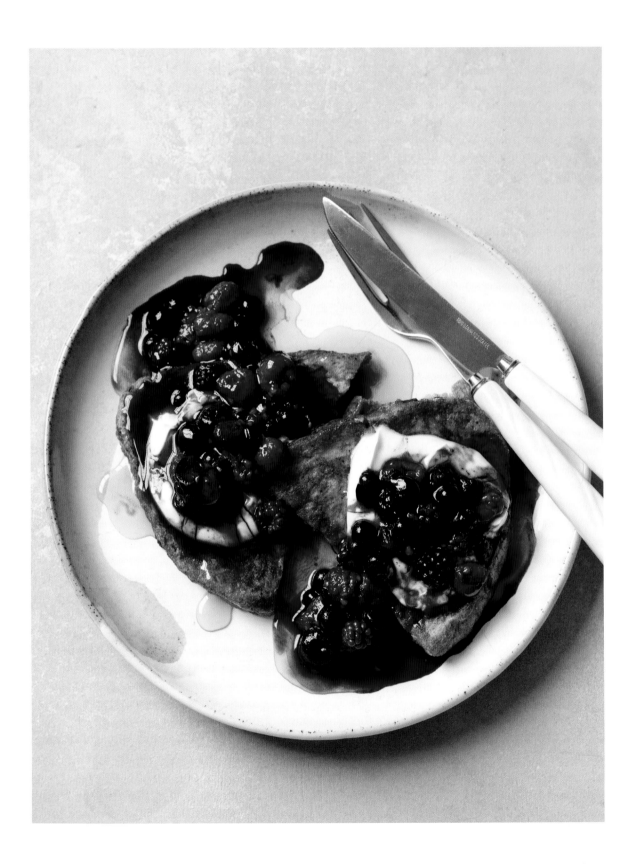

FRENCH TOAST

🍴 serves 2

👨‍🍳 10 mins   ⏱ 5 mins

This is such a warm and delicious breakfast. The cinnamon adds a bit of winter flavor, and the coconut milk makes them nice and sweet—just like me! The topping, made with maple syrup, yogurt and berries, always leaves me wanting more.

Calories: 400 kcal · Carbohydrates: 38 g · Fat: 20 g · Protein: 14 g

2 eggs
⅓ cup + 1 tablespoon coconut milk, or other milk of your choice
1 teaspoon vanilla extract
1 teaspoon ground cinnamon
2 slices of stale whole wheat bread, cut in half diagonally
1 tablespoon coconut oil

Topping:
2 tablespoons coconut yogurt
2½ cups frozen berries, defrosted (or use fresh)
4 teaspoons maple syrup

1. Place the eggs in a shallow bowl with the milk, vanilla and cinnamon and beat to combine thoroughly. Dip the triangles of bread in the mixture, covering both sides and allowing it to soak in.

2. Heat the coconut oil in a large frying pan over medium heat. Lay the triangles of bread in the pan and fry for a few minutes on each side, or until golden brown.

3. Serve hot with the yogurt, berries and maple syrup.

⤷ SWAP

Vegan Use 1 tablespoon of ground chia seeds instead of the eggs and let the mixture activate in the refrigerator for 10 minutes before dipping the bread into it.

BANANA PROTEIN PANCAKE STACK

serves 2

10 mins

20–25 mins

This is a delicious and nutritious breakfast or brunch. The chia seeds add a lovely texture and an extra bit of protein; the protein powder is optional, but it does add a nice flavor—you could even try chocolate protein powder. I love making pancakes on the weekend for friends or just for myself, and these are so quick and easy to make. Serve them with a drizzle of maple syrup, some fresh berries or even a dollop of peanut butter.

Calories: 382 kcal · Carbohydrates: 45 g · Fat: 14 g · Protein: 16 g

1 scoop of vanilla protein powder (optional)
1 ripe banana
¼ cup milk of your choice (I like coconut milk)
1½ cups rolled oats

½ teaspoon ground cinnamon
2 tablespoons chia seeds
½ teaspoon baking powder
pinch of salt
2 large eggs
light cooking oil spray

Serving suggestions:
maple syrup
fresh berries
peanut butter

1. Place all the ingredients, except the oil, in a blender or food processor and blend until smooth.

2. Heat a small frying pan over low heat, spray lightly with oil and spoon in one-sixth of the mixture to make a pancake. Cook for about 2 minutes, then flip and cook on the other side until golden. Repeat to make 6 pancakes in all.

3. Arrange 3 pancakes in a stack on a plate for each serving.

4. Place any leftover pancakes in an airtight container and store in the refrigerator for up to 7 days. Reheat in the toaster before serving.

FRITTATA

🍴 serves 2, generously

👨‍🍳 10 mins   ⏱ 25–30 mins

A frittata makes a nutritious and protein-packed breakfast—it is a perfectly balanced way to start your day. You can make your frittatas in batches and keep them in the refrigerator for breakfast on the go— they taste great hot or cold.

Calories: 478 kcal · Carbohydrates: 22 g · Fat: 30 g · Protein: 31.4 g

1 tablespoon olive oil, plus extra for greasing
1 onion, finely sliced
1 garlic clove, chopped
¾ cup frozen peas
10 cherry tomatoes, halved

6½ cups fresh or frozen spinach, defrosted
handful of chopped fresh herbs, such as parsley or thyme
finely grated zest and juice of **1** lemon

salt and pepper
⅓ cup goat cheese, sliced
6 eggs, beaten

Serving suggestion: green salad

1. Preheat the oven to 400°F (200°C), and grease an ovenproof dish.

2. Heat the olive oil in a frying pan over medium heat, add the onion and garlic and cook for about 5 minutes or until the onion softens. Add the peas and tomatoes and cook for a further minute.

3. Add the spinach, herbs, lemon zest and juice and season well with salt and pepper. Cook for another minute or two until the spinach has wilted.

4. Arrange the veggies evenly over the bottom of the prepared ovenproof dish and place the goat cheese slices over the top. Pour over the eggs and bake for 20 minutes, or until just set. Cut into squares and serve hot or cold with a green salad.

↪ SWAP

Vegan Use a vegan cheese instead of goat cheese and swap the eggs for a chickpea batter. In a large bowl, mix 1½ cups of chickpea flour (gram flour) with 1½ cups of water and 1 tablespoon of olive oil to make the batter. Season with a pinch of salt and pepper and pour over the veggies in place of the eggs.
Fish Swap the goat cheese for 3.5 ounces smoked salmon slices for a fish-themed dish.

BRUNCH SALAD OF DREAMS

🍴 serves 2, generously

👨‍🍳 15 mins, plus cooling   ⏱ 35 mins

I love having my salad of dreams on a Sunday. Chopping and tossing the salad is so relaxing, and I find a salad at breakfast is really refreshing. If I make it on a Sunday, I usually keep a portion for Monday's breakfast or lunch—it's a great way to meal prep. This is balanced and nutritious, just the way I like it!

Calories: 733 kcal · Carbohydrates: 59 g · Fat: 40 g · Protein: 26 g

1⅔ cups sweet potatoes, scrubbed and cut into wedges
15-ounce can chickpeas, rinsed and drained
1 tablespoon olive oil
salt
2 teaspoons *ras el hanout* (Moroccan spice blend)
1 avocado, sliced
10–15 cherry tomatoes, halved
½ red onion, sliced

handful of mint leaves, chopped
3 cups baby spinach leaves
2 hard-boiled eggs, halved
1 tablespoon pumpkin seeds
1 tablespoon sunflower seeds
pepper

Dressing:
3 pitted dates, soaked in hot water for 5 minutes

2 teaspoons extra-virgin olive oil
¼ cup apple cider vinegar
1 teaspoon yellow or grain mustard
¾-inch piece of fresh root ginger, peeled and chopped
1 garlic clove, peeled
pinch of ground cinnamon

1. Preheat the oven to 400°F (200°C), and line a baking sheet with parchment paper.

2. Spread the sweet potatoes and chickpeas out on the lined baking sheet, drizzle with the olive oil and sprinkle with salt and the ras el hanout. Toss to coat, then cook for 30–35 minutes until tender. Set aside to cool.

3. To make the dressing, drain the dates, reserving the water, and place in a blender or food processor with 3 tablespoons of the soaking water and all the other dressing ingredients. Blend until smooth, then season with salt and pepper to taste. If you'd like the dressing a little thinner, add a little more of the soaking water and blend again.

4. Put all the other salad ingredients, apart from the eggs and seeds, in a serving bowl and toss together. Add the cooled sweet potatoes and chickpeas. Top with the eggs, scatter the seeds over the top and season with pepper. Serve with the dressing.

⤷ **SWAP**

Fish/meat Swap the chickpeas for 3.5 ounces of flaked, cooked salmon or 1 sliced, cooked chicken breast. Add the salmon or chicken to the salad just before serving.

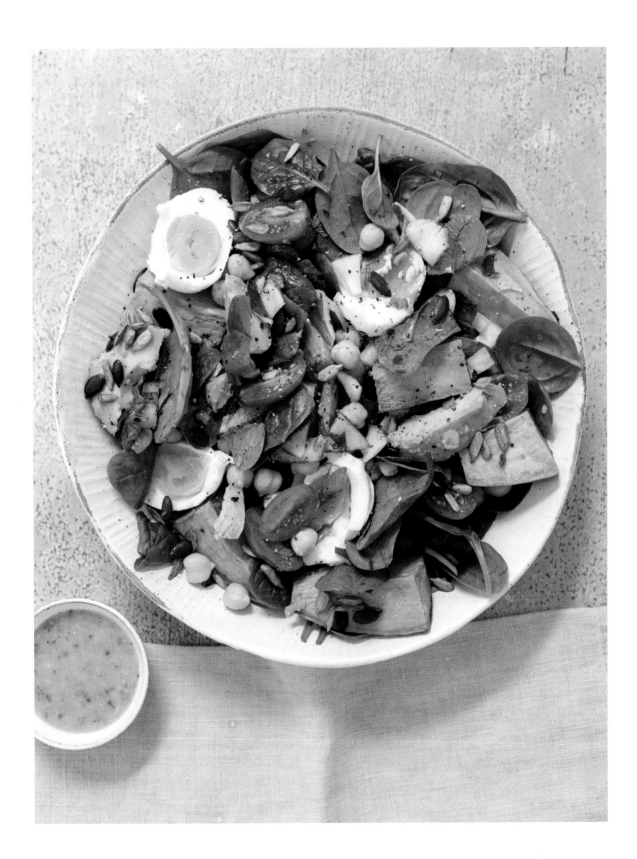

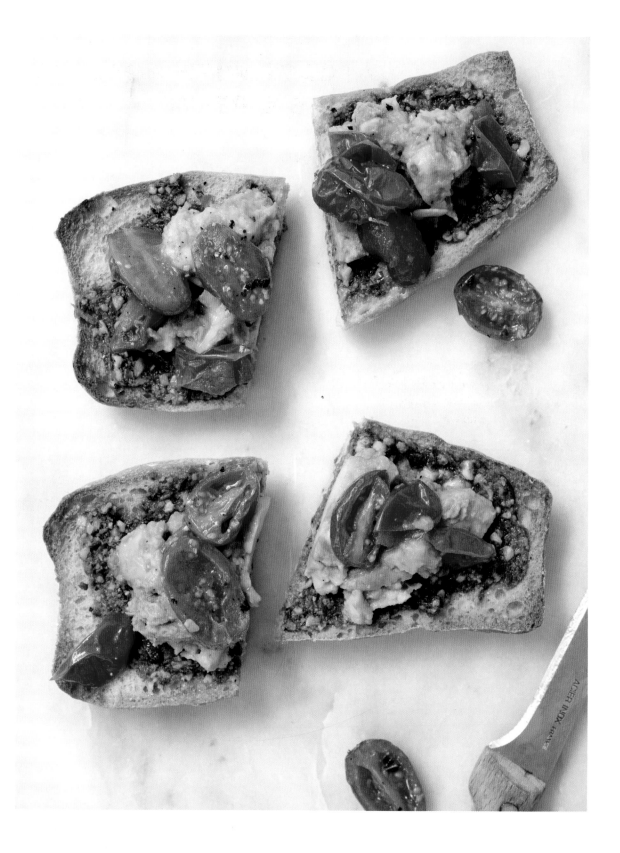

SMASHED AVO TOAST WITH ROASTED TOMATOES & PESTO

serves 2

10 mins   10 mins

I bet you thought bruschetta was just a starter, right? Wrong! This is a really nice way to have your toast in the morning. The olive oil and pesto keep you fueled all morning, giving you the energy you need to have a productive start to the day. I hope you love it.

Calories: 361 kcal · Carbohydrates: 23.5 g · Fat: 25.5 g · Protein: 7 g

10 cherry tomatoes, halved
1 tablespoon olive oil
salt and pepper
1 ripe avocado

squeeze of lemon juice
2 teaspoons pesto
2 slices of toasted ciabatta

1. Preheat the oven or grill to 400°F (200°C). Place the cherry tomatoes and half the olive oil in an ovenproof dish, toss well to coat and season with salt and pepper. Cook for 10 minutes, or until softened.

2. Scoop the avocado flesh into a small bowl, smash with the back of a fork and add the remaining olive oil, the lemon juice and a pinch of salt.

3. Spread the pesto onto the toast, then load the smashed avocado and roasted tomatoes on top.

✒ TIP
This topping would work just as well on rice cakes for a quick, simple brunch.

BREAKFAST BUDDHA BENTO

¶¶ serves 2

👨‍🍳 **15 mins**   ⏱ **35 mins**

Just like a traditional bento box, this delicious meal contains so many flavors and textures and is packed with all your key nutrients too. Save this one for a morning when you want to have a bit of fun in the kitchen or for a home-cooked brunch with friends.

Calories: 769 kcal · Carbohydrates: 63 g · Fat: 43 g · Protein: 27 g

Kale salad:
¾ cup quinoa or brown rice (or a mixture of both)
1 cup kale, stalks removed, chopped
½ teaspoon sea salt
1 tablespoon olive oil, plus extra to drizzle
juice of **1** lime

Roasted sweet potatoes:
2 small sweet potatoes, scrubbed and cut into about ¾-inch chunks
½ tablespoon olive oil
1½ teaspoons salt

2 tablespoons Easy Hummus (see page 92)
1 small avocado, sliced
2 hard-boiled eggs, halved
1 tablespoon tahini
1 tablespoon mixed seeds or nuts

1. Cook the quinoa in a saucepan of lightly salted boiling water for about 15 minutes until tender, then drain and set aside to cool.

2. Meanwhile, preheat the oven to 400°F (200°C), and line a baking sheet with parchment paper.

3. Place the sweet potatoes in a large bowl with the olive oil and salt and toss until coated. Spread out on the lined baking sheet and cook for 30–35 minutes, or until tender. Set aside to cool.

4. Place the kale in a large bowl. Sprinkle with the salt and drizzle with a little olive oil. Use your hands to massage the kale for 2–3 minutes to soften it.

5. Whisk the tablespoon of olive oil and the lime juice together in a bowl, drizzle over the kale and toss to coat. Add the cooled quinoa and toss together.

6. Divide the kale salad and roasted sweet potatoes between 2 bento boxes and add the hummus, avocado and eggs. Drizzle the tahini over the top and sprinkle with seeds or nuts. Put the lids on and keep cool until you are ready to eat.

☑ TIP
For some extra spice, toss the sweet potato in 1 teaspoon of smoked paprika and 2 teaspoons of ground cumin with the olive oil and salt.

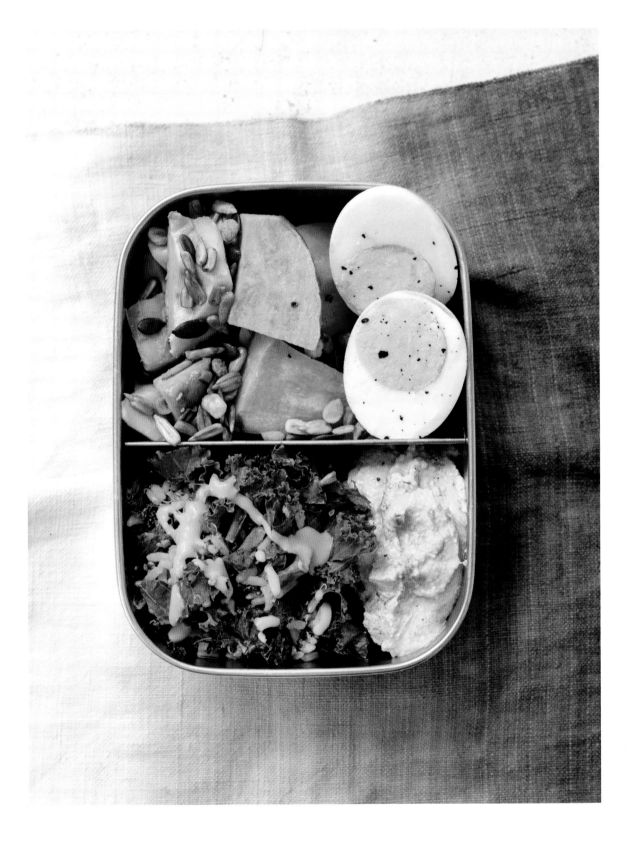

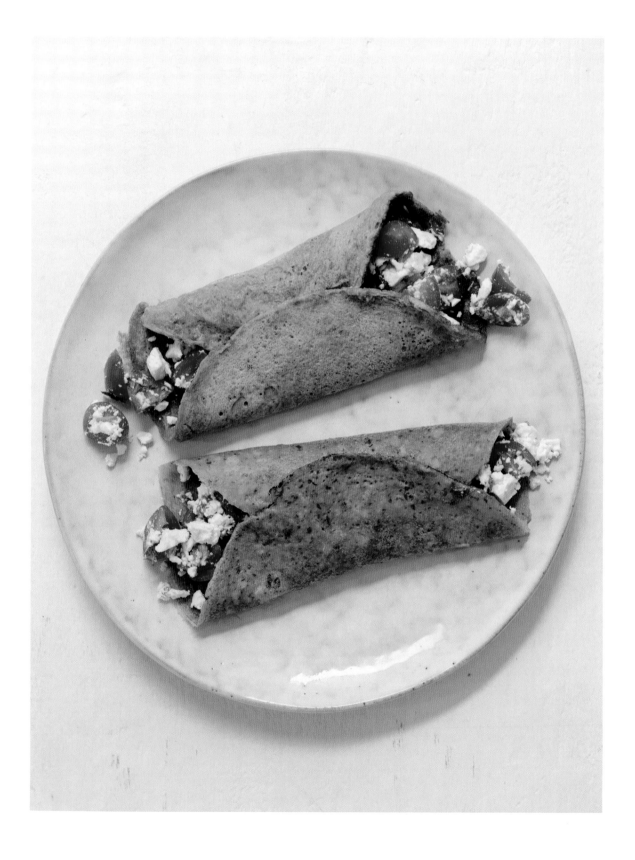

SPINACH & FETA CRÊPES

⑪ serves 2

👨‍🍳 **5 mins**　　　　　⏱ **15 mins**

Who said crêpes are just for dessert? I love savory crêpes, especially for breakfast. These are so filling and a great way to get some veggies in the morning. I make a batch of the crêpes without the filling and keep them in the refrigerator or freezer for a quick breakfast another day. I'm always planning ahead!

Calories: 447 kcal · Carbohydrates: 53 g · Fat: 15 g · Protein: 20 g

1¼ cups plain wholemeal flour
3 cups spinach leaves
1 large egg
1 cup almond milk, or other
milk of your choice
salt and pepper
olive oil, for frying

Filling:
3 tablespoons feta cheese,
crumbled
small handful of parsley,
chopped
8 cherry tomatoes,
quartered

1. Put the flour, spinach, egg and milk in a blender or food processor, season well with salt and pepper and blend thoroughly until smooth.

2. Heat a large frying pan over medium heat. Drizzle in a tiny amount of olive oil, then pour in one-quarter of the crêpe batter, tilting the pan to spread it evenly. Cook for about 1 minute, then flip the crêpe over or turn using a spatula.

3. Arrange one-quarter of the feta, parsley and tomatoes along the center of the crêpe, then fold over the edges to enclose the filling. Cook for 1 more minute, then transfer to a plate and keep warm.

4. Repeat to make 4 crêpes in total. Serve 2 crêpes per person.

⤷ **SWAP**

Vegan Swap the egg for ½ cup of chickpea flour (gram flour) and use 1 tablespoon of nutritional yeast instead of the feta cheese.

SMOKY BEANS & GREENS ON TOAST

serves 4, generously

10 mins　　　　　　**15 mins**

This is my version of traditional beans on toast, which I loved as a kid and used to have at school too. By adding a variety of spices and vegetables, I now enjoy it as a nutritious and balanced breakfast. It keeps me fueled right through to lunch, and I love it.

Calories: 468 kcal · Carbohydrates: 63.3 g · Fat: 17.4 g · Protein: 15.7 g

4 tablespoons olive oil
2 onions, thinly sliced
4 garlic cloves, chopped
4 teaspoons smoked paprika
1 teaspoon crushed red pepper
salt and pepper
2 cups kale, stems removed, sliced

15-ounce can cannellini or butter beans, rinsed and drained
half of 14.5-ounce can diced tomatoes
2 tablespoons soy sauce
½ cup + 1 tablespoon water
8 slices of bread (I like rye), toasted

1. Heat the olive oil in a large saucepan over medium heat. Add the onions and garlic and cook for 3–5 minutes until softened. Add the paprika and crushed red pepper and season well with salt and pepper.

2. Add the kale and cook, stirring, until wilted. Now add the beans, chopped tomatoes, soy sauce and measured water. Turn up the heat and simmer for 5 minutes until piping hot. Serve the beans and greens on toast.

3. Any leftover beans and greens can be stored in the refrigerator for up to 3 days, or in the freezer for 3 weeks.

✎ TIP

For extra flavor and protein, chop 3 smoked slices of bacon and add to the pan with the onion and garlic.

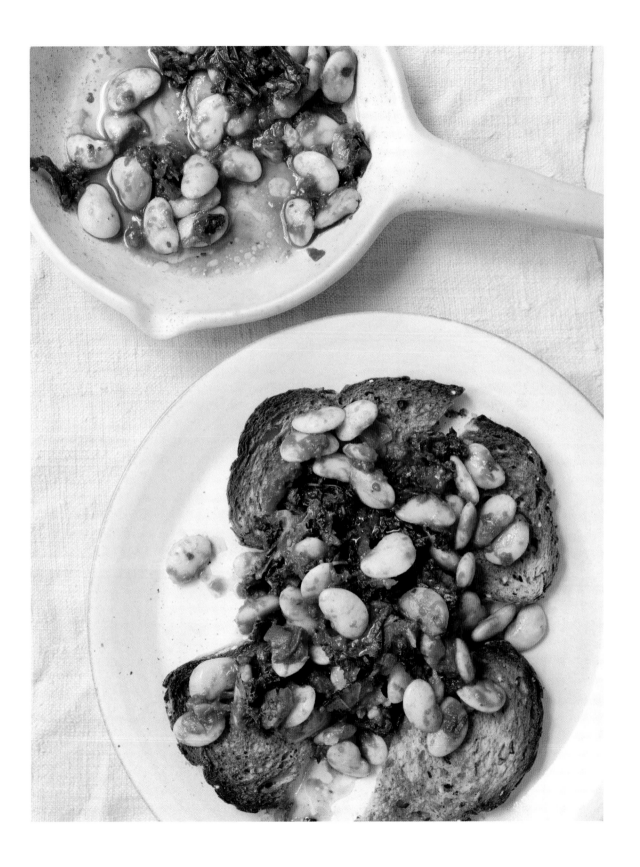

RAINBOW WRAP

🍴 serves 2
👨‍🍳 15 mins

This is such a delicious breakfast to throw together, a creative twist on the traditional breakfast with eggs. My rainbow wraps will make you feel like you're on vacation, and with a few of your own added extras, such as bacon or turkey, you can create your perfect breakfast. These can be wrapped up (literally!) and eaten on the go.

Calories: 375 kcal · Carbohydrates: 27.8 g · Fat: 26.2 g · Protein: 11.3 g

2 small tortilla wraps
2 teaspoons pesto
1 avocado, mashed
handful of baby
    spinach leaves

2 large tomatoes, sliced,
    or 8 cherry tomatoes,
    halved (or a mixture of
    both)
2 hard-boiled eggs, sliced

drizzle of olive oil
squeeze of lemon juice
salt and pepper

1. Lay the wraps on a clean surface and spread with the pesto, then the mashed avocado.

2. Arrange the spinach, tomato and egg on top. Drizzle with a little olive oil and a squeeze of lemon juice and season with salt and pepper.

3. Roll the wraps tightly and serve straight away, or wrap in plastic wrap or foil and keep cool until you are ready to eat.

↪ SWAP

Meat To make this a BLT wrap, swap the egg for 2 grilled slices of bacon per wrap.

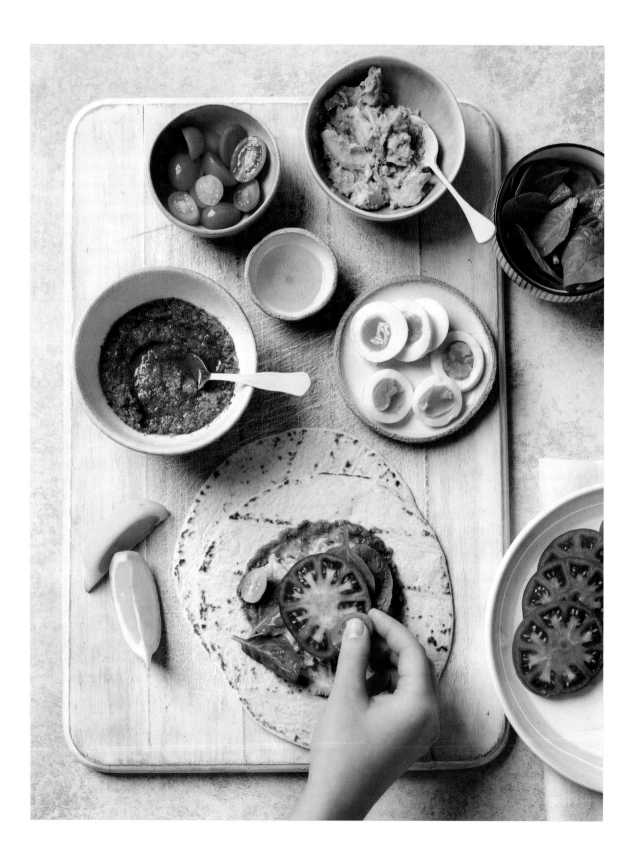

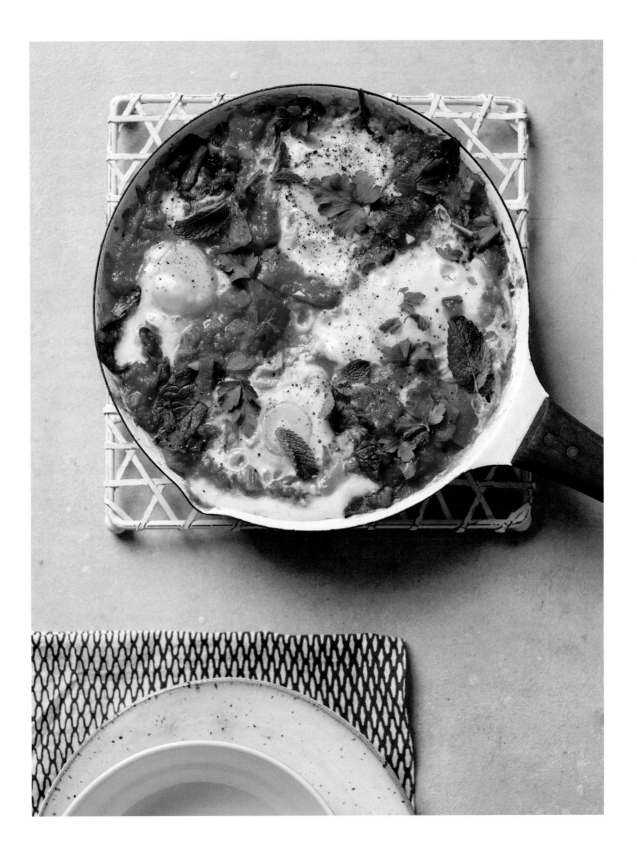

SHAKSHUKA

¶¶ serves 2, generously

👨‍🍳 10 mins   ⏱ 30 mins

I remember when I first tried *shakshuka* and couldn't believe it was a breakfast dish! I love eggs, and I absolutely love my nutritious and wholesome twist on this recipe. I usually have it for breakfast, but if I'm working from home, I sometimes have it for lunch too—it's the perfect amount of food to keep me fueled and energized.

Calories: 300 kcal · Carbohydrates: 35.4 g · Fat: 11.7 g · Protein: 18.2 g

1 tablespoon olive oil
1 onion, chopped
2 peppers, cored, deseeded and chopped
2 garlic cloves, chopped
1 teaspoon smoked paprika

1 teaspoon ground cumin
pinch of crushed red pepper
salt and pepper
4 large tomatoes, chopped
14.5-ounce can diced tomatoes

3 cups spinach leaves
4 large eggs

To garnish:
handful of parsley leaves
handful of mint leaves

1. Heat the olive oil in a large frying pan over medium heat and add the onion, peppers and garlic. Stir in the paprika, cumin and crushed red pepper and season well with salt and pepper. Cook gently, stirring occasionally, for about 10 minutes or until softened.

2. Add the fresh and canned tomatoes and stir thoroughly. Bring to a boil, cover and simmer gently for 15 minutes, then remove the lid and cook for a few minutes more until thickened. Stir in the spinach.

3. Make 4 holes in the sauce with a spoon and break the eggs into them. Cover the pan again and cook gently for a few minutes until the egg whites are set and the yolks are still runny. Sprinkle over the herbs and serve.

⤷ SWAP

Vegan Swap the eggs for a 15-ounce can of chickpeas, rinsed and drained, adding the chickpeas to the pan with the tomatoes.
Meat Fry 7 ounces of extra-lean ground beef or lamb in a little olive oil until browned, season well with salt and pepper and add to the pan with the tomatoes.

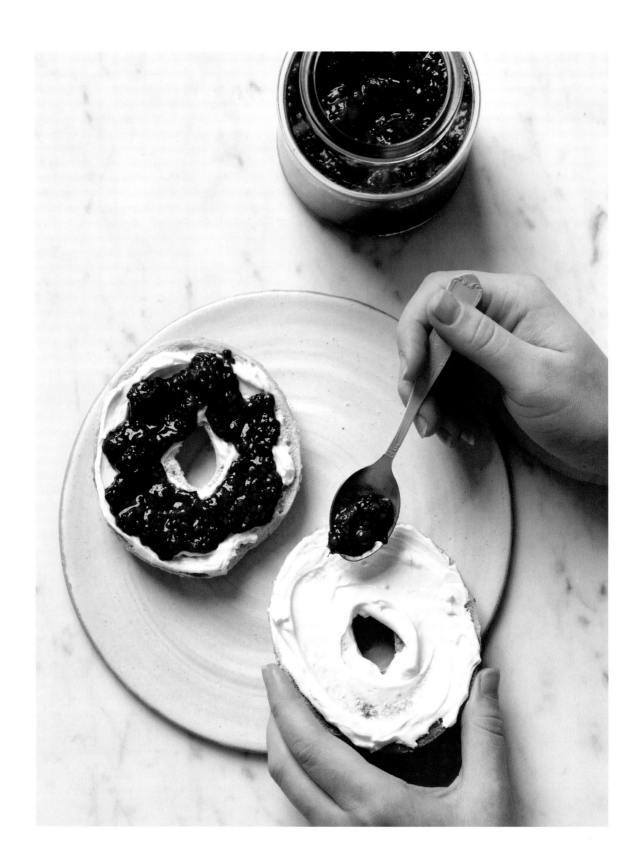

A BAGEL A DAY

Bagels are life! They're delicious, and can be eaten with your favorite toppings. From chocolate to cheese—not at the same time!—I've created mouth-watering options for you. They'll have you jumping out of bed for breakfast.

CHIA JAM & CREAM CHEESE BAGEL

🍴 serves 1, with leftover jam

👨‍🍳 5 mins, plus cooling   ⏱ 15 mins

I highly recommend making some of this protein-rich jam to keep in the refrigerator for a speedy breakfast or snack. Just spread it on toast, bagels or rice cakes. It tastes amazing, trust me! You can use any berries for this, so feel free to experiment—frozen raspberries are my favorite.

> ♡ Bagel plus topping
>
> **Calories:** 590 kcal · **Carbohydrates:** 102.3 g · **Fat:** 16.6 g · **Protein:** 15 g

- **1¾ cups** fresh or frozen berries
- **1 tablespoon** lemon juice
- **1 tablespoon** honey or maple syrup
- **2 tablespoons** chia seeds
- **2 tablespoons** water
- **1 tablespoon** cream cheese
- **1** bagel, split and toasted

1. Place the berries in a saucepan over medium heat, crushing with a fork and stirring until the liquid is bubbling and the fruit has softened.

2. Stir in the lemon juice, honey or maple syrup, chia seeds and measured water, remove from the heat and allow to cool. The jam will thicken as it cools.

3. To serve, spread the cream cheese over a toasted bagel and top with one-sixth of the jam.

4. Store the leftover jam in an airtight jar in the refrigerator for up to 2 months.

🖊 TIP
For added flavor and nutrition, top your bagel with sliced strawberries.

CHOCOLATE & HAZELNUT SPREAD BAGEL

¶¶ serves 1, with leftover spread

👨‍🍳 15 mins, plus cooling   ⏱ 15 mins

Here's your very own chocolate and hazelnut spread recipe, and it tastes so good! Having a jar in my refrigerator for my toast, bagels or simply a sneaky spoonful is just my favorite. It's so easy to put together with so few ingredients— let me know what you think, but be sure not to finish the whole jar in one sitting. I usually serve this with sliced banana on top.

♡ Bagel plus topping

Calories: 527 kcal · Carbohydrates: 19.6 g · Fat: 48.1 g · Protein: 11.3 g

2½ cups unsalted hazelnuts
½ cup dark chocolate, broken into pieces
1 teaspoon vanilla extract
pinch of salt

1 teaspoon maple syrup (optional)
1 bagel, split and toasted

Serving suggestion:
1 banana, sliced

1. Preheat the oven to 325˚F (160˚C). Spread the hazelnuts out on a baking sheet and cook for 8–10 minutes until golden, keeping an eye on them to prevent burning. Allow to cool slightly.

2. Place the hazelnuts in a blender or food processor and blend on low speed for about 8 minutes, scraping down the sides every so often, until very smooth.

3. Meanwhile, place the chocolate in a heatproof bowl over a small saucepan of gently simmering water, making sure the water does not touch the bowl. Stir occasionally until melted.

4. Once the hazelnut butter is smooth, add the vanilla and salt and blend to combine. Add the melted chocolate and blend again until well mixed. Taste and add the maple syrup to sweeten, if using.

5. To serve, spread one-sixth of the spread over a toasted bagel. Top with sliced banana, if you fancy.

6. Store the leftover spread in an airtight jar for up to 4 weeks.

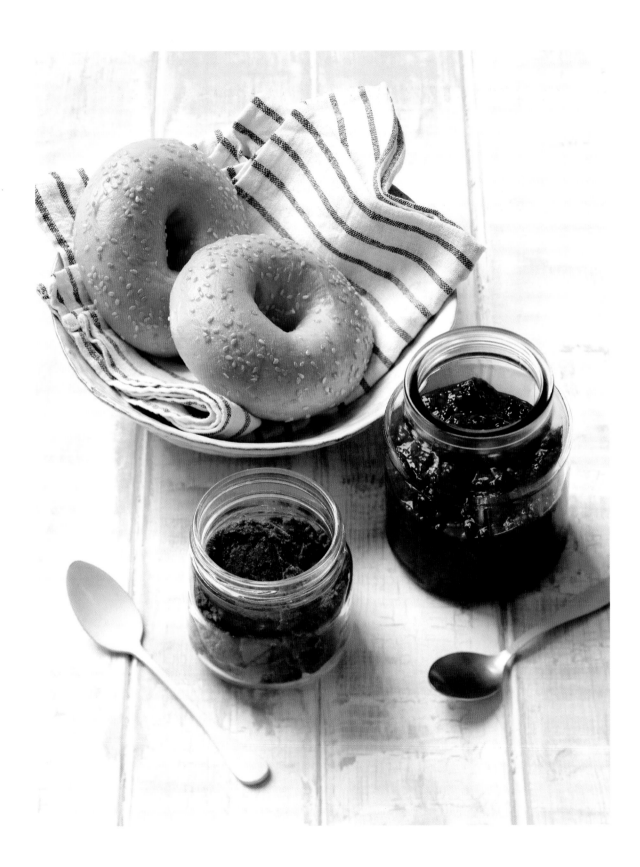

CARROT LOX BAGEL

Ⅱ serves 1, with leftover carrot lox
⌂ 15 mins, plus cooling and marinating   ⏱ 1 hour

This is a delicious vegan version of lox, the traditional Jewish dish of cured salmon. I would recommend making this when you have a bit of time in your schedule, and keep any leftovers for snacks. The carrots taste lovely on bagels—I really love this topping!

♡ Bagel plus topping

Calories: 549 kcal · Carbohydrates: 86.9 g · Fat: 15.8 g · Protein: 16.8 g

---

3 large carrots, scrubbed
coarse rock salt, for sprinkling
1 tablespoon olive oil
1 teaspoon smoked paprika
splash of soy sauce

juice of **1** lemon
1 bagel, split and toasted
1 tablespoon cream cheese
chopped fresh dill, to garnish

---

1. Preheat the oven to 400°F (200°C). Place the damp carrots in a small ovenproof dish and sprinkle liberally with rock salt. Cook, uncovered, for 1 hour.

2. When the carrots are cool enough to handle, crack away or brush off the salt, then peel away the skins using a sharp knife. Slice the carrots into thin slices lengthways using a mandoline or sharp knife and place in an airtight container.

3. Whisk the olive oil, paprika, soy sauce and lemon juice together in a bowl, drizzle over the warm carrots and toss well to coat. Cover and place in the refrigerator overnight to marinate.

4. The next morning, allow the carrots to come to room temperature. Spread the toasted bagel with the cream cheese and top with one-sixth of the carrots and a sprinkling of fresh dill.

5. Store any leftover carrot lox in the refrigerator for up to 7 days.

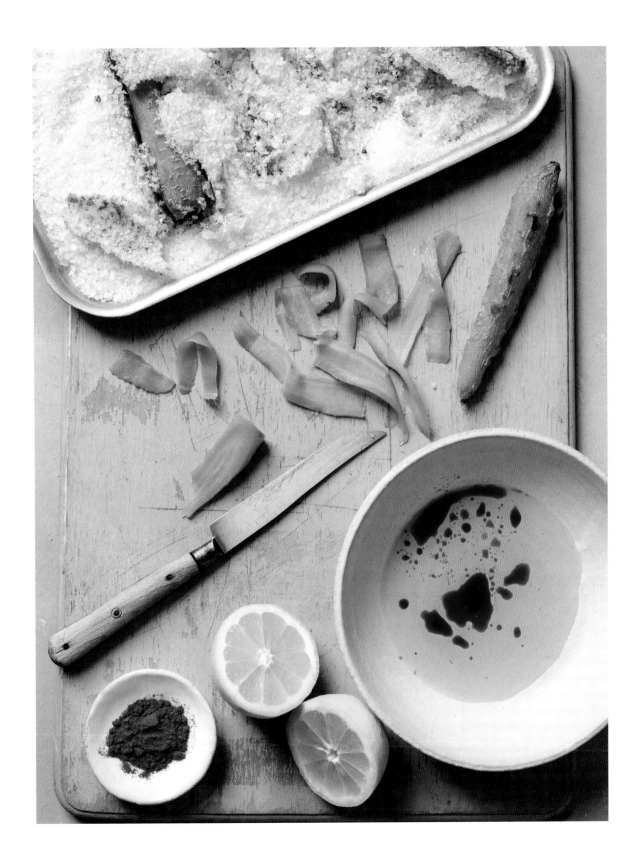

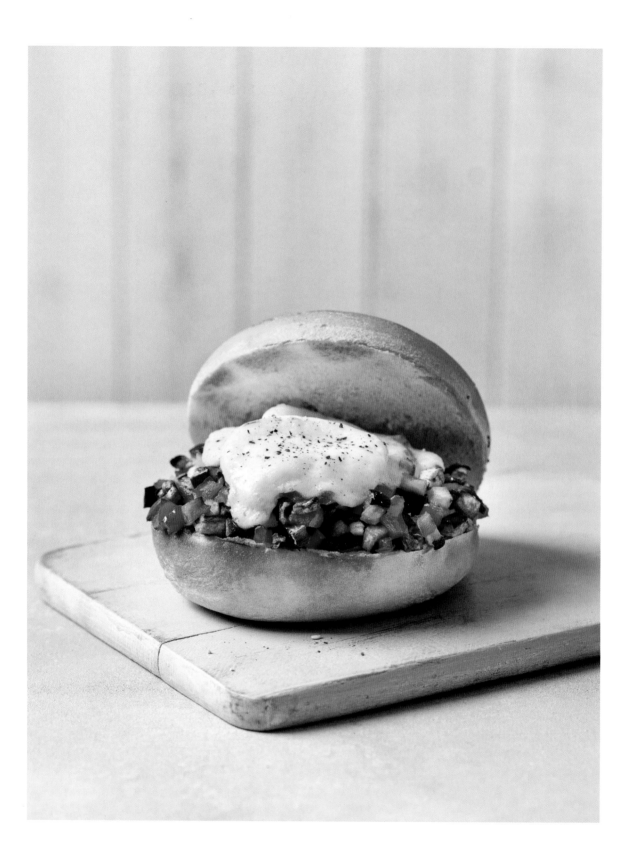

GRILLED VEGGIE BAGELS
WITH MOZZARELLA

🍴 serves 2

👨‍🍳 10 mins　　　⏱ 25 mins

This is the perfect weekend breakfast! I've created a bagel topping that adds so many vegetables into your diet in the morning. The maple syrup provides the most delicious flavor. This is another great recipe to make if you have company, and it works for lunch too.

♡ Bagel plus filling

Calories: 516 kcal · Carbohydrates: 83 g · Fat: 15.7 g · Protein: 14.6 g

2 tablespoons olive oil

1 red pepper, cored, deseeded and finely chopped

1 red onion, finely chopped

1 zucchini, sliced

1 eggplant, finely chopped

1 garlic clove, unpeeled

1 tablespoon maple syrup

salt and pepper

2 bagels, split and toasted

¼ cup mozzarella cheese, sliced

1. Preheat the oven to 400°F (200°C), and drizzle the olive oil over a baking sheet. Spread the vegetables and garlic on the baking sheet and drizzle with the maple syrup. Season well with salt and pepper and toss to coat in the oil and syrup. Cook for 20 minutes, or until tender and golden, turning once.

2. Pile the veggies onto 2 toasted bagel halves, return to the baking tray and top with the mozzarella. Cook for a further 5 minutes, or until the cheese has melted. Serve topped with the remaining toasted bagel halves.

ULTIMATE BREAKFAST BAGEL

¶¶ serves 2

👨‍🍳 **15 mins**   ⏱ **20 mins**

This bagel makes you feel like you're having a burger for breakfast—my mouth waters just thinking about it! It's so simple to put together and so tasty. Feel free to get creative with this one and substitute the bacon for tofu, or try turkey slices instead. And if you're feeling like something extra, add some grilled veggies and mozzarella cheese (see page 73).

> ♡ Bagel plus filling
> Calories: 740 kcal · Carbohydrates: 49.8 g · Fat: 39.8 g · Protein: 44.3 g

4 slices of bacon
4 slices of Halloumi cheese
2 bagels, split
2 tablespoons olive oil
2 eggs

1 beefsteak tomato, sliced
sweet chili sauce, to serve
chopped fresh chives, to
  garnish

1. Place the bacon in a frying pan over medium heat and cook, turning once, until golden and crispy. Transfer to a plate, then add the Halloumi to the pan and fry in the bacon fat, turning once, until golden. Set aside with the bacon.

2. Preheat the grill to medium and toast the bottom halves of the bagels on both sides until golden.

3. Enlarge the holes in the top halves of the bagels until big enough to hold the eggs.

4. Heat the olive oil in the frying pan over medium heat and add the top halves of the bagels, cut side down. Crack the eggs into the holes in the bagels

and cook for a minute or so until the eggs have set on the bottom. Place the frying pan under the grill until the egg whites are just cooked and the bagels are golden.

5. Place the bottoms of the bagels on 2 plates and top with sliced tomato. Add the bacon and Halloumi, then add a dollop of sweet chili sauce. Garnish with the chives, and finish with the bagel tops with eggs in them and enjoy.

➔ SWAP
Veggie Replace the bacon with slices of smoked tofu, frying until lightly golden.

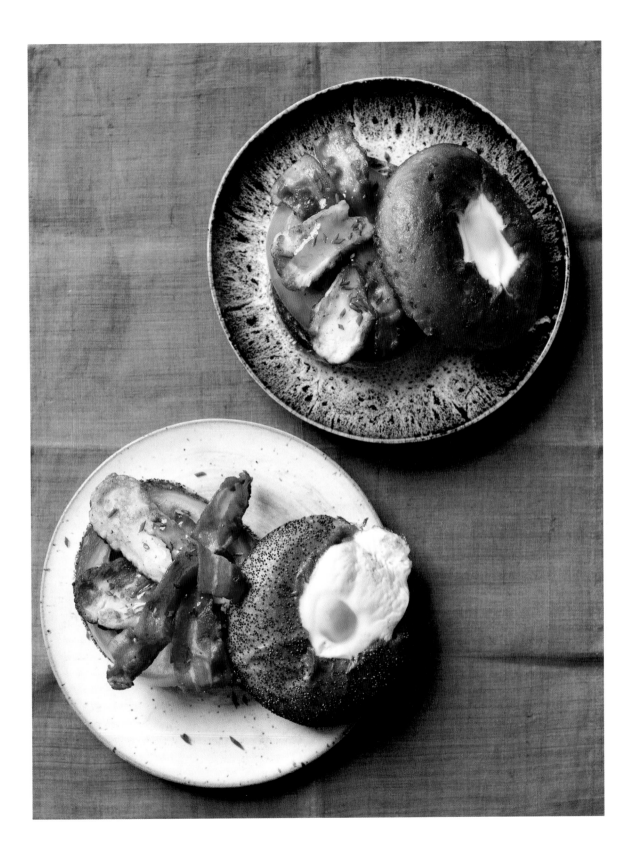

SNACKS

MINI OMELETTES

makes 12 omelettes

10 mins   **15 mins**

I love eggs, and they're a great source of protein too. These omelettes are so simple to make, and you can pretty much add any of your favorite vegetables, herbs or spices to them. They're also great for breakfast if you're in a rush.

Calories: 76 kcal · Carbohydrates: 1.3 g · Fat: 4.7 g · Protein: 5.6 g

olive oil, for greasing
1½ cups baby spinach leaves, finely shredded
1 small red onion, thinly sliced
6 pitted black olives, sliced

1½ tablespoons cooked ham, chopped (optional)
8 eggs, beaten
salt and pepper
½ cup feta cheese, crumbled

1. Preheat the oven to 400°F (200°C), and grease a 12-hole nonstick muffin pan with olive oil.

2. Divide the spinach, onion, olives and ham, if using, between the holes in the pan. Season the eggs with salt and pepper and pour into the holes in the pan, then crumble the feta over the top. Cook for 15 minutes, or until golden brown.

3. Leave to cool for 5 minutes in the pan, then transfer to a wire rack to cool completely.

4. Any leftover omelettes can be stored in an airtight container in the refrigerator for up to 5 days.

TROPICAL AMAZEBALLS

🍴 **makes 10 balls**
👨‍🍳 **10 mins**

Energy balls are really convenient and can be stored in the freezer—so easy! For you fruit lovers, I've created some sunny tropical ones that actually make you feel like you're on the beach. If you don't like coconut, simply leave it out.

Calories: 167 kcal · Carbohydrates: 18 g · Fat: 9.2 g · Protein: 2.4 g

1 cup walnuts
¾ cup pitted dates, soaked in hot water for 5 minutes (reserve the water)
½ cup dried papaya
1 tablespoon coconut oil

1 tablespoon rolled oats
1 tablespoon honey or maple syrup
2 tablespoons shredded coconut, plus extra for coating

1. Place the walnuts in a food processor and chop for 30 seconds. Add the drained dates and papaya and mix for another 30 seconds, then add the coconut oil, oats and honey or maple syrup and mix for 2 minutes. Add a little of the date soaking water if the mixture is very dry, then add the shredded coconut and mix for another minute. If you don't have a food processor, you can use a blender, loosening the mixture with a little warm water, if necessary.

2. Roll the mixture into 10 even-sized balls, about 1 inch in diameter, then roll them in a little more shredded coconut to coat.

3. Store in an airtight container in the refrigerator for up to 7 days, or in the freezer for up to 3 months.

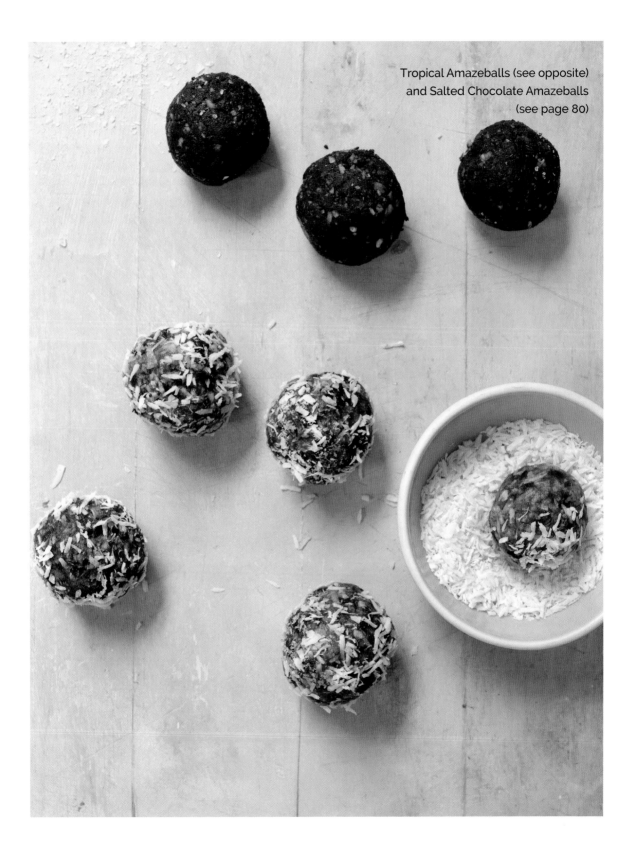

Tropical Amazeballs (see opposite) and Salted Chocolate Amazeballs (see page 80)

SALTED CHOCOLATE AMAZEBALLS

🍴 makes 10 balls

🎩 10 mins

These taste delicious, and I love carrying a few with me, especially when I'm commuting and get hungry.

Calories: 160 kcal · Carbohydrates: 16 g · Fat: 8.8 g · Protein: 3.2 g

1 cup walnuts

1½ cups pitted dates, soaked in hot water for 5 minutes (reserve the water)

1 tablespoon coconut oil

1 tablespoon rolled oats

1 tablespoon honey or maple syrup

1 tablespoon cocoa powder, plus extra for coating

1 tablespoon rock salt

1. Place the walnuts in a food processor and chop for 30 seconds. Add the drained dates and mix for another 30 seconds, then add the coconut oil, oats and honey or maple syrup and mix for 2 minutes. Add a little of the date soaking water if the mixture is very dry, then add the cocoa and salt and mix for another minute. If you don't have a food processor, you can use a blender, loosening the mixture with a little warm water, if necessary.

2. Roll the mixture into 10 even-sized balls, about 1 inch in diameter, then roll them in a little more cocoa to coat.

3. Store in an airtight container in the refrigerator for up to 7 days, or in the freezer for up to 3 months.

PRETZELS WITH PEANUT BUTTER & CHOCOLATE

🍴 serves 2

👨‍🍳 10 mins, plus freezing   ⏱ 5 mins

These pretzels will make your mouth water—smothered in peanut butter and melted dark chocolate, they taste amazing! Make a batch and just snack on them anytime. They take next to no time to prep and are great when you've got friends around or fancy a movie night.

Calories: 294 kcal · Carbohydrates: 33.5 g · Fat: 15.5 g · Protein: 12.5 g

1 tablespoon peanut butter
1 cup pretzel twists
⅓ cup dark chocolate, broken into pieces

1. Line a plate with parchment paper.

2. Use a knife to spread the peanut butter over the pretzel twists so it fills the holes.

3. Place the chocolate in a heatproof bowl over a small saucepan of gently simmering water, making sure the water does not touch the bowl. Stir occasionally until melted.

4. Dip the pretzels, one at a time, into the melted chocolate and spread out on the parchment paper. Place in the freezer for 20 minutes to harden and then enjoy.

5. Any leftovers can be stored in an airtight container in the refrigerator or freezer for up to 3 weeks.

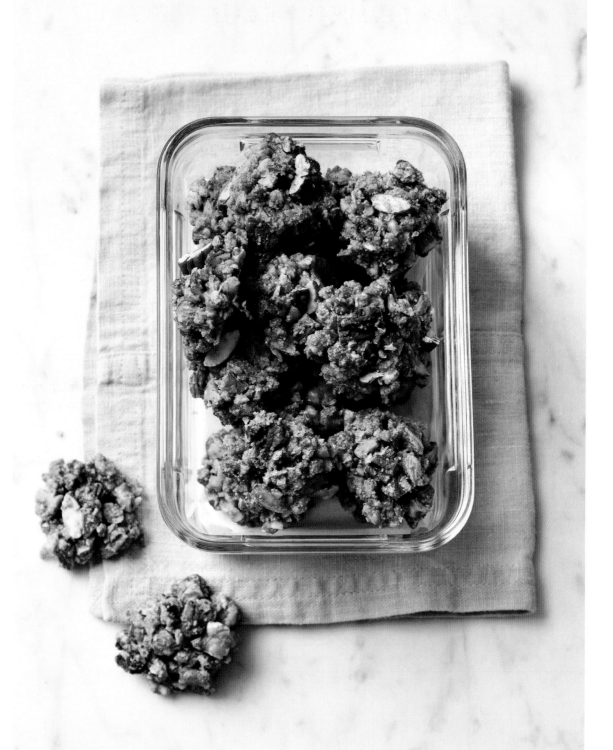

SALTED NUT CLUSTERS

♔ makes 20 clusters

👨‍🍳 10 mins   **⏱ 20 mins**

These nut clusters are delicious, have so much flavor and make the perfect savory snack to stop you from feeling hungry. Prep takes no time at all, and once they're ready, you can keep them in an airtight container to nibble on. But be careful, you'll end up eating all the clusters before you know it.

Calories: 85 kcal · Carbohydrates: 4 g · Fat: 7.5 g · Protein: 2 g

¾ cup almonds, roughly chopped
¾ cup walnuts, roughly chopped
¾ cup pecans, roughly chopped
½ cup ground almonds

1 teaspoon ground cinnamon (optional)
1 teaspoon sea salt, plus extra for sprinkling
3 tablespoons maple syrup

1. Preheat the oven to 325°F (160°C), and line a baking sheet with parchment paper.

2. Place all the ingredients in a large bowl and mix well. Drop 20 portions (2 teaspoons each) of the mixture onto the lined baking tray, spacing them out evenly. Cook for about 20 minutes until golden. Leave to cool and harden on the baking tray, then sprinkle with a little more salt.

3. Store in an airtight container for up to 4 weeks.

SWEET POTATO TOASTS

🍴 makes 4 toasts

👨‍🍳 5 mins   ⏱ 15–20 mins

I had so much fun combining different flavors to top my sweet potato toasts. Filled with so many nutrients, these are great to have after a workout. Make the sweet potato toasts in advance so that when you're hungry, you'll have a delicious snack in no time.

Calories: 28 kcal · Carbohydrates: 6.5 g · Fat: 0 g · Protein: 5 g

1 sweet potato, scrubbed

1. Preheat the oven to 350°F (180°C), and line a baking sheet with parchment paper.

2. Trim the pointed ends from the sweet potato and then slice it lengthways into ¼-inch slices using a sharp knife. You will get about 4 slices from a medium sweet potato.

3. Lay the slices on the lined baking tray and cook for 15–20 minutes until tender. Allow to cool.

4. Store in an airtight container in the refrigerator for up to 3 days, or in the freezer for 3 weeks.

5. When you are ready to eat, place a sweet potato toast into a toaster or toaster oven. Toast until piping hot with crispy edges. Add your choice of topping.

PEANUT & BANANA TOPPING

🍴 serves 1   👨‍🍳 5 mins

♡ **Sweet Potato Toast plus topping**
Calories: 143 kcal · Carbohydrates: 27.7 g · Fat: 3 g · Protein: 2.9 g

1 tablespoon peanut butter
½ banana, sliced

AVOCADO & EGG TOPPING

🍴 serves 1   👨‍🍳 10 mins

♡ **Sweet Potato Toast plus topping**
Calories: 287 kcal · Carbohydrates: 22.1 g · Fat: 19.4 g · Protein: 8.6 g

---

½ avocado, mashed
1 hard-boiled egg, sliced

COTTAGE CHEESE & CHIVE TOPPING

🍴 serves 1   👨‍🍳 5 mins

♡ **Sweet Potato Toast plus topping**
Calories: 71 kcal · Carbohydrates: 13.5 g · Fat: 0.6 g · Protein: 2.6 g

---

1 tablespoon cottage cheese
sprinkling of snipped chives

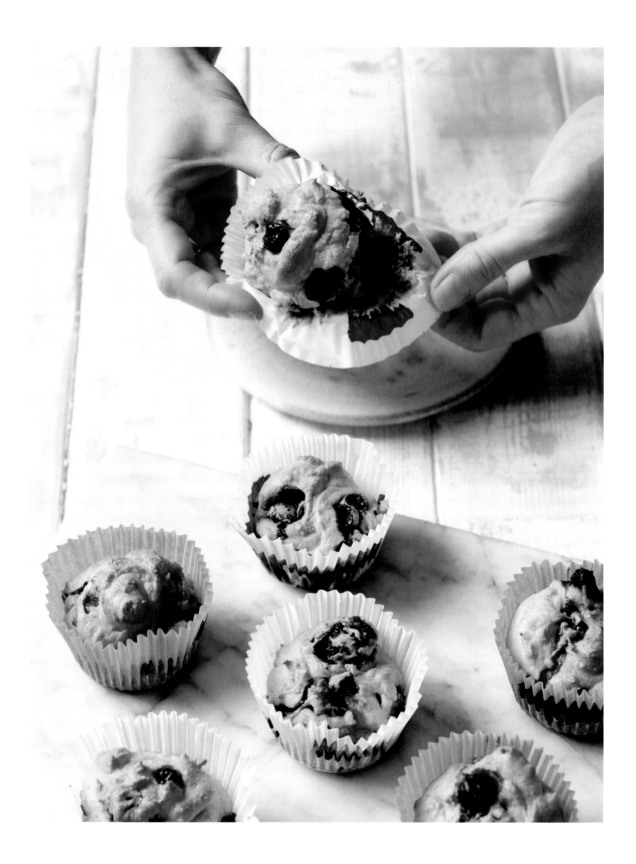

PROTEIN BLUEBERRY MUFFINS

makes 8 muffins

10 mins   **15 mins**

I love blueberry muffins, and I've created a great post-workout snack version.
These are perfect with tea or coffee, or take one to work as your afternoon snack.

Calories: 94 kcal · Carbohydrates: 12 g · Fat: 3.1 g · Protein: 5.3 g

1¼ cups oat flour or rolled
   oats
1 scoop of vanilla protein
   powder
1 teaspoon baking powder
½ cup Greek yogurt

1 teaspoon vanilla extract
1 egg
¼ cup almond milk, or other
   milk of your choice
½ cup blueberries

1. Preheat the oven to 375°F (190°C),
and line 8 holes of a muffin pan with paper liners.

2. If using rolled oats, blend them in a blender or
food processor until they resemble flour.

3. Place the oat flour in a large bowl and add the
protein powder and baking powder.

4. Place the yogurt, vanilla, egg and milk in a bowl
and whisk thoroughly. Pour into the dry ingredients
and mix well. Add the blueberries and fold in gently.

5. Divide the mixture between the muffin cups and
cook for about 15 minutes until they have risen well
and bounce back when pressed. Transfer to a wire
rack to cool.

6. Store in an airtight container for up to 3 days,
or in the freezer for up to 3 weeks.

POST-WORKOUT SNACKS

TUNA RICE CAKES

🍴 serves 1   👨‍🍳 5 mins

With more protein than Rice Cakes with Smashed Avo (see page 99), these are perfect after a workout.

Calories: 190 kcal · Carbohydrates: 13 g · Fat: 1.8 g · Protein: 30 g

5-ounce can tuna in water, drained
juice of **½** lemon
½ teaspoon paprika

salt and pepper
2 rice cakes
cucumber slices, to serve

1. Mash the tuna in a bowl with the lemon juice and paprika and season with salt and pepper to taste.

2. Spread the tuna mixture over the rice cakes and serve with sliced cucumber.

STUFFED AVO WITH COTTAGE CHEESE

🍴 serves 1   👨‍🍳 5 mins

This is a quick-and-easy vegetarian snack with protein to fuel you after you've just smashed your workout. It's a nice way to liven up an avocado if you have one that needs eating—we usually do!

Calories: 249 kcal · Carbohydrates: 12 g · Fat: 20 g · Protein: 8 g

¼ cup low-fat cottage cheese
salt and pepper

½ ripe avocado
a few walnuts, chopped

1. Season the cottage cheese with salt and pepper and spoon into the hole in the avocado.

2. Sprinkle with walnuts and some extra pepper.

CHILI SALTED EDAMAME BEANS

🍴 serves 1　　👨‍🍳 5 mins

I love devouring these after a workout. Edamame beans can be bought shelled or in the pod. If yours are in the pod, simply slip them out into a bowl.

Calories: 141 kcal · Carbohydrates: 11.1 g · Fat: 6.4 g · Protein: 12.4 g

¾ cup cooked edamame beans
½ teaspoon rock salt

pinch of garlic powder
pinch of crushed red pepper

1. Mix the beans with the seasonings in a small bowl and tuck in.

SMASHED CHICKPEA DIP

🍴 serves 3　　👨‍🍳 5 mins

This is a nice source of protein after a workout. Serve this dip with veggie crudités or spread it on rice cakes.

Calories: 57 kcal · Carbohydrates: 6.7 g · Fat: 2.5 g · Protein: 2.4 g

15-ounce can chickpeas, rinsed
and drained
finely grated zest and juice
of **1** lemon

pinch of crushed red pepper
pinch of salt
pinch of smoked paprika
drizzle of olive oil

1. Place all the ingredients in a bowl and mash with the back of a fork or a potato masher to make a coarse paste.

2. Store in an airtight container in the refrigerator for up to 5 days.

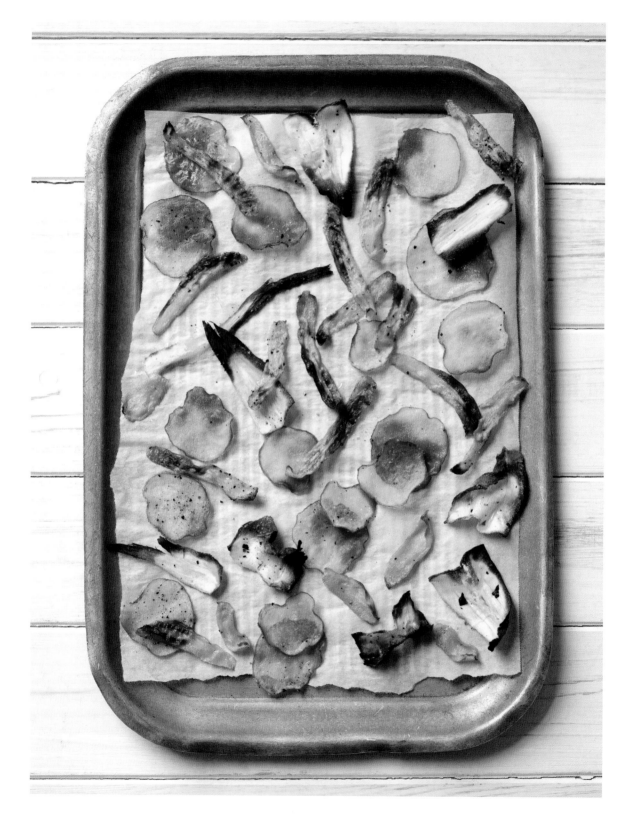

HOME-BAKED SALTED CHIPS

¶¶ serves 3

👨‍🍳 10 mins   ⏱ 10 mins

I make these if I've got friends coming over, and it helps me use up all the vegetables in my refrigerator! Once you've got all the chopping out of the way, they are so easy to cook, and they're a tasty way of getting your extra veggies in. These chips are best eaten the day they are made, so if you don't need three servings, reduce the quantities accordingly.

Calories: 223 kcal · Carbohydrates: 33.2 g · Fat: 9.3 g · Protein: 3.4 g

1 large carrot, peeled
1 large parsnip, peeled
1 large potato, peeled

2 tablespoons olive oil
2 teaspoons salt
black pepper

1. Preheat the oven to 400°F (200°C), and line a baking sheet with parchment paper.

2. Slice the veggies very thinly on a mandoline, being careful of your fingers. Alternatively, a sharp knife will do the job.

3. Dry the slices very thoroughly on a clean tea towel, one vegetable at a time, and transfer the vegetables to a mixing bowl. Pour the oil into the bowl and combine very well to coat, then arrange the veggies in a single layer on the lined baking sheet. Season well with salt and pepper.

4. Cook for 6–8 minutes until the vegetables are golden and cooked through, removing them from the baking sheet when they are ready—the carrots may cook a little more quickly than the others. Season again and allow to cool.

EASY HUMMUS

serves 6
5 mins

If I could eat hummus all day, I would—and I do eat it most days. I have it on toast or on a rice cake to fuel my day. I love the flavors of paprika and cumin—they give it a nice kick! Serve on brown toast with an extra squeeze of lemon and add a fried egg if you wish.

Calories: 98 kcal · Carbohydrates: 0.3 g · Fat: 5.1 g · Protein: 3.4 g

15-ounce can chickpeas, rinsed and drained
juice of **1** lemon
1 tablespoon tahini
1 small garlic clove, chopped

2 tablespoons olive oil
1 teaspoon ground cumin
1 teaspoon paprika
½ cup water
salt

1. Place all the ingredients in a blender or food processor and blend on high speed for a few minutes until smooth, adding a little more water if it looks too dry.

2. Store in an airtight container in the refrigerator for up to 3 days.

SMOKED MACKEREL PÂTÉ

🍴 serves 6
👨‍🍳 10 mins

Full of protein, this pâté is so easy to prepare and wonderful with toast. Keep some in the refrigerator for a convenient snack. This would work really well after a workout too. I like to serve it on brown toast or a rice cake, topped with snipped watercress and a squeeze of lemon juice.

Calories: 212 kcal · Carbohydrates: 2 g · Fat: 18.5 g · Protein: 9.5 g

9 ounces smoked mackerel fillets, skinned
finely grated zest and juice of **1** lemon
⅔ cup cream cheese
handful of parsley leaves
2 tablespoons creamed horseradish
pepper

1. Place all the ingredients in a blender or food processor and blend until smooth, or leave it a little chunkier if you prefer.

2. Store in an airtight container in the refrigerator for up to 3 days.

FRUIT & NUT CHOC COOKIES

🍴 **makes 10 cookies**

👨‍🍳 **10 mins**   ⏱ **10 mins**

I need to have cookies with my coffee or tea, and I love baking these. They're filled with everything I love, and my friends and family can't stop eating them either. You could double the quantities to make extra cookie dough to freeze and bake at a later date.

Calories: 205 kcal · Carbohydrates: 27 g · Fat: 8.6 g · Protein: 3.5 g

1¾ cups oat flour or rolled oats
pinch of salt
½ teaspoon baking powder
½ cup brown sugar
⅓ cup dark chocolate, chopped
⅓ cup raisins

½ cup almonds or walnuts, chopped
1 teaspoon vanilla extract
2 tablespoons melted coconut oil
½ cup milk of your choice (I like coconut milk)

1. Preheat the oven to 375°F (190°C), and line a baking sheet with parchment paper.

2. If using rolled oats, blend them in a blender or food processor until they resemble flour.

3. Place all the dry ingredients in a mixing bowl and stir well to combine. Place the vanilla, coconut oil and milk in a bowl and whisk with a fork, then add to the dry ingredients and mix well to form a ball of dough.

4. Shape the dough into 10 even-sized balls and arrange, well spaced, on the lined baking sheet. Bake for 8–10 minutes, until golden. Leave to cool on a wire rack.

5. Store in an airtight container for up to 3 days.

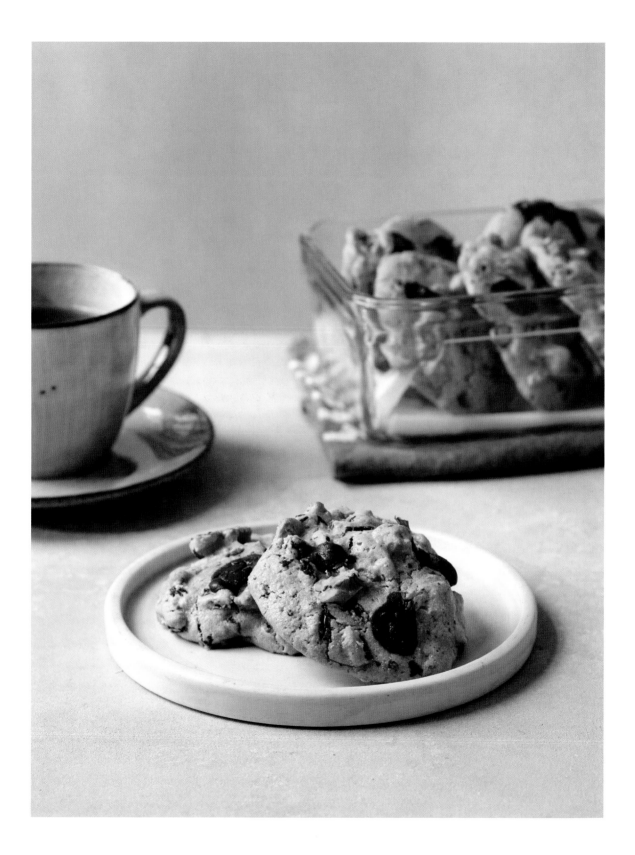

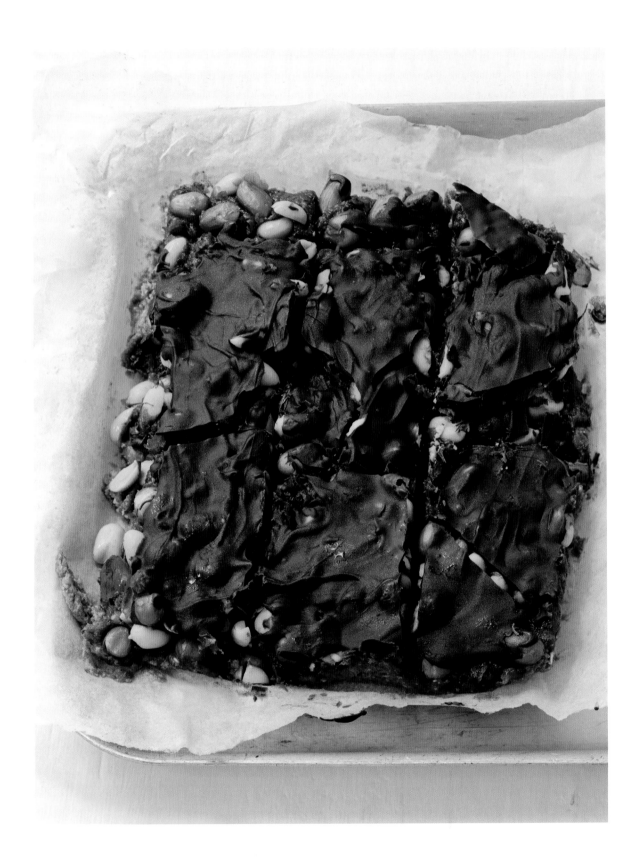

PEANUT CARAMEL CHOCOLATE BAR

makes 9 bars

20 mins, plus freezing   **5 mins**

I had so much fun making my very own chocolate bar, and it tastes delicious. This is a great snack and one you can make in batches to keep in your cupboard—thank me whenever you have a sweet craving!

Calories: 214 kcal · Carbohydrates: 31 g · Fat: 9.3 g · Protein: 4.3 g

Caramel:
1¼ cups pitted dates, soaked in hot water for 5 minutes
2 tablespoons peanut butter

1 teaspoon vanilla extract
1 teaspoon salt

¾ cup oat flour or rolled oats
¼ cup salted peanuts
½ cup dark chocolate, broken into pieces

1. Line a large plate and an 8-inch square brownie pan with parchment paper.

2. If using rolled oats, blend them in a blender or food processor until they resemble flour.

3. To make the caramel, drain the dates and place in a blender or food processor with all the other caramel ingredients. Blend until thick and smooth, making sure you scrape down the sides so you don't waste any. Transfer the caramel to a bowl.

4. To make the base layer, place the oat flour in the blender (no need to rinse) with 3 tablespoons of the date caramel and blend until it resembles a sticky dough. Firmly press the mixture into the bottom of the lined pan in an even layer.

5. Use a spatula to spread the remaining caramel over the base, then sprinkle the peanuts evenly over the top, pressing them into the caramel so they stick. Place in the freezer for 1 hour.

6. Place the chocolate in a heatproof bowl over a small saucepan of gently simmering water, making sure the water does not touch the bowl. Stir occasionally until melted.

7. Carefully pour the melted chocolate over the frozen mixture. Return to the freezer for 30 minutes, then use a sharp knife to cut the mixture into 8 even bars.

8. Transfer to an airtight container and store for up to 3 days.

SPEEDY SNACKS

APPLE & PEANUT BUTTER

🍴 serves 1   👨‍🍳 5 mins

The peanut butter in this snack provides protein to satisfy hunger, and the apple adds sweetness—perfect for when you're feeling a bit peckish.

Calories: 191 kcal · Carbohydrates: 28.7 g · Fat: 8.6 g · Protein: 4.1 g

1 apple
1 tablespoon peanut butter

1. Core and cut the apple into chunky wedges. Spread the peanut butter evenly over the slices, or use it as a dip.

SLICED SPICED BANANA

🍴 serves 1   👨‍🍳 5 mins

Bananas are a great source of potassium, fiber and protein.

Calories: 175 kcal · Carbohydrates: 26 g · Fat: 5.3 g · Protein: 3.8 g

1 banana
½ tablespoon nut butter (any nut butter will work)
1 teaspoon honey
ground cinnamon, for sprinkling

1. Slice the banana and arrange the slices on a small plate. Top each slice with a little nut butter. Drizzle the honey on top and sprinkle with a little ground cinnamon, to taste.

STUFFED DATES

🍴 serves 1   👨‍🍳 5 mins

I absolutely love dates—this snack makes it feel like Christmas.

Calories: 166 kcal · Carbohydrates: 19.5 g · Fat: 7.5 g · Protein: 1.6 g

pinch of ground cinnamon
2 teaspoons nut butter (any nut butter will work)
2 pitted Medjool dates

1. Mix the ground cinnamon into the nut butter. Use it to stuff the dates.

RICE CAKES WITH SMASHED AVO

🍴 serves 1   👨‍🍳 5 mins

I always have rice cakes at home—I can add pretty much anything to them.

Calories: 216 kcal · Carbohydrates: 16 g · Fat: 17 g · Protein: 2.5 g

½ avocado
pinch of crushed red pepper
pinch of salt

juice of ½ lime
drizzle of olive oil
1 rice cake

1. Mash together the avocado flesh, crushed red pepper, salt, lime juice and olive oil. Spread on a rice cake.

MISO BROTH

🍴 serves 1   👨‍🍳 5 mins

Miso is a fermented food, so it's great for your gut. This broth is really comforting.

Calories: 25 kcal · Carbohydrates: 3 g · Fat: 0.5 g · Protein: 2 g

1 tablespoon miso paste

1. Stir the miso paste into a mug of hot water and enjoy.

LUNCH

STUFFED PEPPERS

¶¶ serves 2, generously

🎩 **15 mins**   ⏱ **30 mins**

Stuffed peppers make a great meal to share with friends and family and are fab for a barbecue too. Top with yogurt, mint and chopped jalapeño, and you're good to go!

Calories: 802 kcal · Carbohydrates: 80 g · Fat: 38.1 g · Protein: 26.4 g

2 red peppers, halved lengthways, cored and deseeded
3 garlic cloves, crushed
1 tablespoon olive oil, plus extra for drizzling
salt and pepper
½ cup brown rice
1 large onion, finely sliced
1 fresh jalapeño, deseeded and finely chopped

2 teaspoons smoked paprika
1 cup sun-dried tomatoes from a jar, drained and chopped
1 teaspoon harissa
finely grated zest and juice of **1** lemon
bunch of parsley, chopped
½ cup walnuts, chopped
½ cup bread crumbs
¼ cup Cheddar cheese, grated

Topping:
½ cup natural yogurt
1 bunch of mint, leaves picked and chopped
1 fresh jalapeño, chopped

Serving suggestion:
mixed green salad

1. Preheat the oven to 400°F (200°C).

2. Score the flesh of the peppers in a criss-cross pattern, leaving the skin intact. Spread the peppers with half the garlic and drizzle with a little olive oil. Season with salt and pepper really well and arrange on a baking sheet. Cook for 20 minutes, or until softened.

3. Meanwhile, cook the rice in a saucepan of lightly salted boiling water according to the packet instructions until tender. Drain and set aside.

4. Heat 1 tablespoon of olive oil in a large saucepan over medium-low heat and add the onion, jalapeño, and remaining garlic. Cook for 5 minutes, or until softened. Stir in the paprika and cook for another

minute. Add the sun-dried tomatoes, harissa, lemon zest and juice, parsley, walnuts and cooked rice and give it a really good mix. Season well.

5. Preheat the grill. Divide the rice mixture between the peppers, packing it in neatly. Top with the bread crumbs, cheese and another drizzle of olive oil. Grill for 5 minutes, or until golden.

6. To serve, drizzle the yogurt over the top and sprinkle with the mint, jalapeño and a little salt. Serve with a mixed green salad.

⤷ SWAP

Vegan Swap the grated cheese for a spoonful of nutritional yeast.

KRISSY SALAD

🍴 serves 2, generously
👨‍🍳 10 mins

My clients often call salads "rabbit food." I always tell them they haven't tried a salad made by yours truly. Salads can be so much fun to make—I actually find all the chopping so enjoyable and feel like I'm a pro-chef tossing it all around in my salad bowl! Obviously this is my favorite salad in the book, but all of them are delicious and make a great lunch or even dinner. You can add your own ingredients too, getting creative with your leafy greens and brightly colored veggies—make your salads just how you like them.

Calories: 504 kcal · Carbohydrates: 37 g · Fat: 31 g · Protein: 16 g

Dressing:
1 tablespoon honey or maple syrup
dash of yellow or grain mustard
3 tablespoons fresh orange juice
1½ tablespoons balsamic vinegar
2 teaspoons extra-virgin olive oil
salt and pepper

4 cooked beets, cut into wedges
⅓ cup goat cheese, sliced
½ cup walnuts, chopped
⅓ cup raisins
handful of chopped parsley
4 cups mixed salad leaves

1. Place all the dressing ingredients in a bowl and whisk to combine. Season to taste.

2. Place all the salad ingredients in a large serving bowl, pour the dressing over and toss thoroughly.

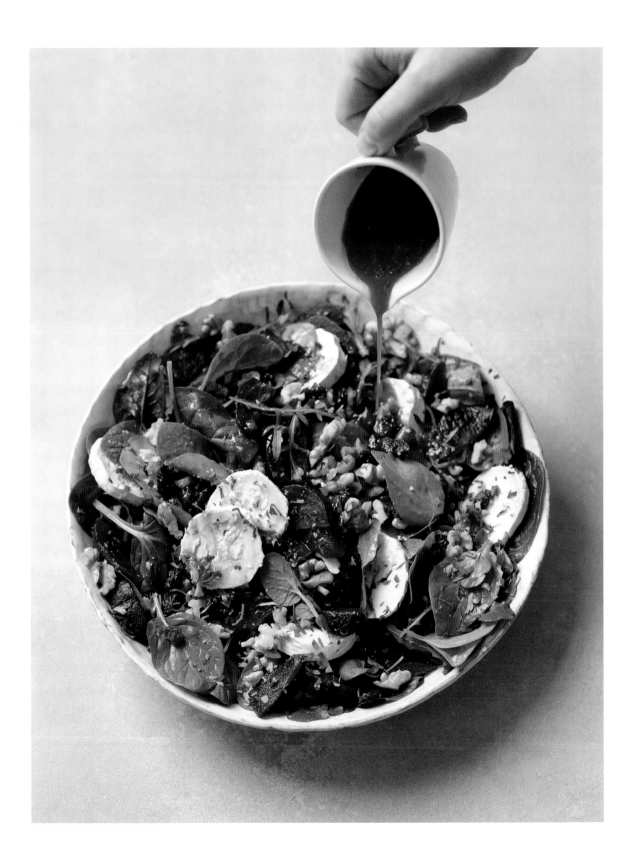

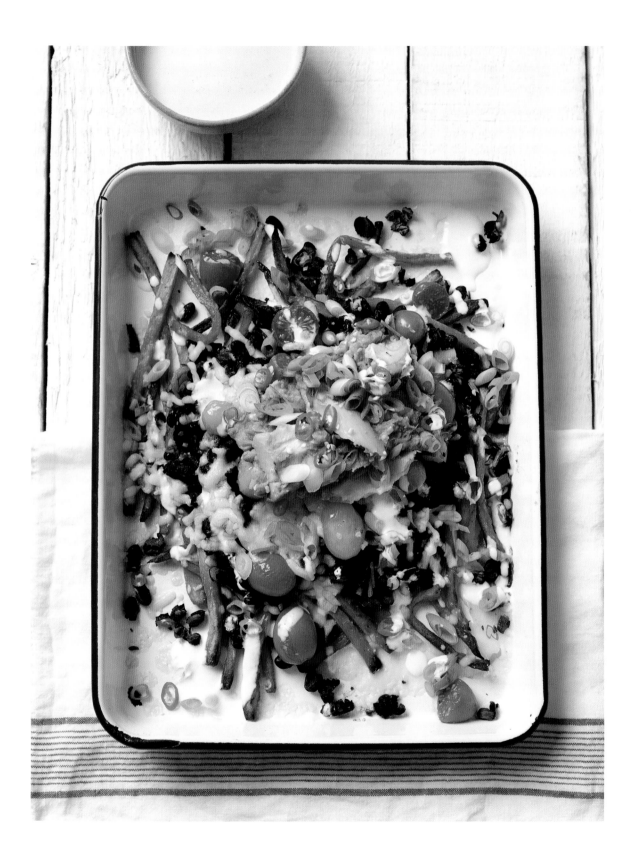

LOADED SWEET POTATO FRIES

¶¶ serves 2, generously

👒 **15 mins**   ⏱ **25 mins**

This is possibly my favorite lunch. My loaded fries make me feel like I'm in a Mexican restaurant with all my best friends—now that's a happy and healthy lunch date! They make a great starter or side if you're hosting dinner—your friends and family won't want to move on to the main course.

Calories: 658 kcal · Carbohydrates: 66 g · Fat: 37.9 g · Protein: 19.2 g

2 tablespoons olive oil
2 sweet potatoes or regular potatoes, cut into ¼-inch wide fries
salt
1 tablespoon reduced-fat sour cream
juice of **1** lime

1 cup black beans, rinsed and drained
10 cherry tomatoes, halved
¼ cup Cheddar cheese, grated
1 avocado, mashed
1 fresh jalapeño, chopped
4 spring onions, sliced

1. Preheat the oven to 400°F (200°C), and line a baking sheet with parchment paper.

2. Heat the olive oil in a large frying pan over medium heat. Add the fries and cook for a few minutes, turning, until they begin to brown. Transfer to the lined baking sheet, season with salt and cook for about 20 minutes until tender and golden.

3. Place the sour cream and lime juice in a small bowl and mix well.

4. Transfer the fries to a large heatproof plate. Top with the beans, cherry tomatoes and cheese and return to the oven for a few minutes until the cheese melts.

5. Top the fries with the sour cream, avocado, jalapeño and spring onions and serve.

SWEET POTATO RÖSTI

🍴 serves 2, generously

👨‍🍳 10 mins   ⏱ 15 mins

Combine the gorgeous flavor of sweet potatoes with a range of tasty toppings and create a wholesome and nutritious meal.

Calories: 314 kcal · Carbohydrates: 44 g · Fat: 11.5 g · Protein: 9 g

1 tablespoon olive oil, plus extra for greasing
3 medium sweet potatoes, peeled
1 small onion, thinly sliced

1 garlic clove, crushed
2 eggs, beaten
salt and pepper

1. Preheat the oven to 425°F (220°C), and lightly grease a nonstick baking sheet.

2. Coarsely grate the sweet potatoes onto a clean tea towel, then collect up the sides of the tea towel and squeeze any excess liquid out of the sweet potatoes. Transfer to a mixing bowl.

3. Heat the oil in a frying pan over medium-low heat, add the onion and garlic and cook for about 5 minutes until softened. Add to the grated potato with the eggs, season well with salt and pepper and mix thoroughly.

4. Divide the mixture into 4 and shape into small cakes. Place on the baking sheet and cook for 20 minutes, or until golden brown. Serve with your choice of topping.

RÖSTI WITH AVOCADO & HUMMUS

🍴 serves 2   👨‍🍳 5 mins

♡ Sweet Potato Rösti plus topping

Calories: 543 kcal · Carbohydrates: 47.7 g · Fat: 32.5 g · Protein: 12.7 g

1 avocado
juice and zest of **2** limes
handful of chopped parsley
2 tablespoons Easy Hummus (see page 92)
1 quantity Sweet Potato Rösti (see above)

1. Chop the avocado, place in a bowl and toss with the lime juice and zest and parsley.

2. Top the rösti with the hummus and the avocado.

RÖSTI WITH HALLOUMI & SWEET CHILI

serves 2   **10 mins**

> ♡ **Sweet Potato Rösti plus topping**
> Calories: 654 kcal · Carbohydrates: 51.4 g · Fat: 35.5 g · Protein: 33 g

olive oil, for frying
8 slices of Halloumi cheese
1 quantity Sweet Potato Rösti (see opposite)
large handful of spinach leaves
sweet chili sauce, to serve

1. Heat a drizzle of olive oil in a frying pan over medium heat, add the Halloumi and cook for about 2 minutes on each side until golden brown.

2. Top the rösti with the spinach leaves and Halloumi, and drizzle with sweet chili sauce.

RÖSTI WITH EGG & ASPARAGUS

serves 2   **10 mins**

> ♡ **Sweet Potato Rösti plus topping**
> Calories: 446 kcal · Carbohydrates: 44.7 g · Fat: 21.5 g · Protein: 17.5 g

olive oil, for frying
2 eggs
1 quantity Sweet Potato Rösti (see opposite)
8 thin asparagus spears
squeeze of lemon juice
salt and pepper

1. Heat a little olive oil in a frying pan. Crack the eggs into the pan and fry for 3 minutes, or until the whites are set. Place the eggs on top of the rösti.

2. Add the asparagus spears to the hot pan and fry for 1 minute, or until golden all over. Squeeze over a little lemon juice and season with salt and pepper, then serve on top of the eggs.

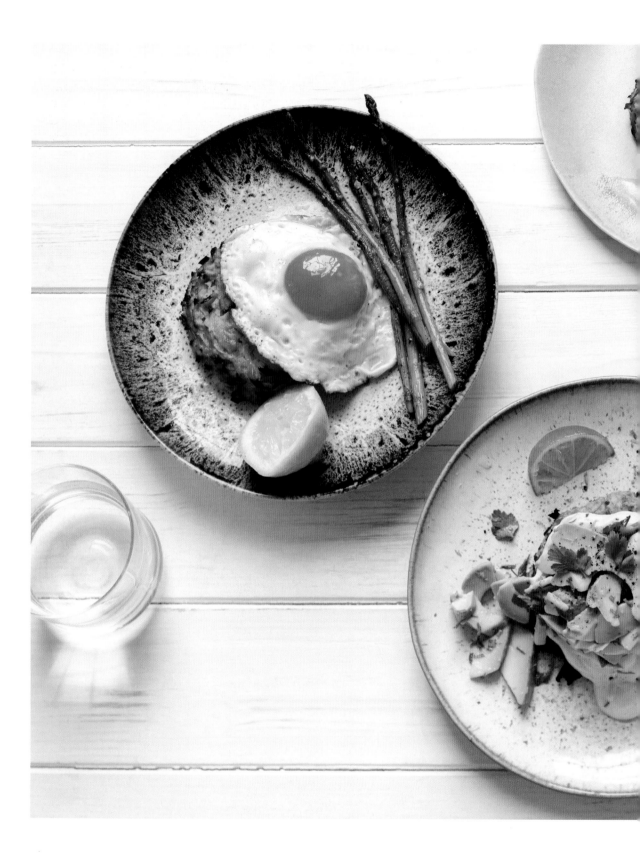

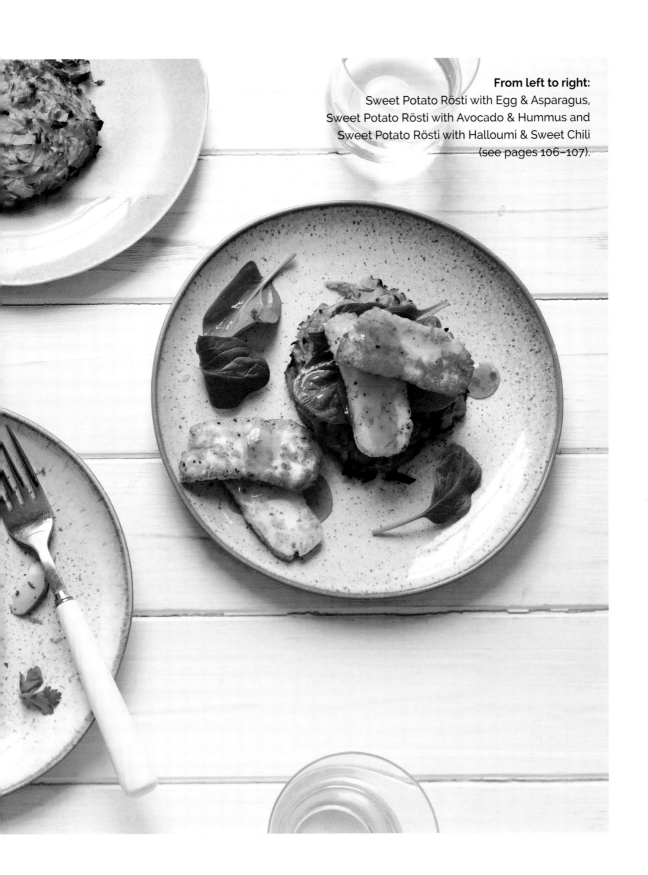

From left to right:
Sweet Potato Rösti with Egg & Asparagus,
Sweet Potato Rösti with Avocado & Hummus and
Sweet Potato Rösti with Halloumi & Sweet Chili
(see pages 106–107).

BUDDHA BOWL

¶¶ serves 2, generously

👨‍🍳 15 mins　　　　　　**⏱ 25 mins**

Buddha bowls are filled with lots of flavor and texture, yet they're so simple to put together. It's easy to include your favorite ingredients, and I just couldn't decide on one style for you, so I've chosen three! Follow the basic recipe to make your Buddha bowl, then choose from one of the three tasty toppings. Feel free to mix and match the ingredients or try out all three and decide which one is your favorite (it's Protein Jalapeño Chicken for me, see page 112).

Calories: 618 kcal · Carbohydrates: 48 g · Fat: 33 g · Protein: 25 g

⅓ cup brown rice or quinoa
1 small avocado, halved
15-ounce can black beans or
　chickpeas, rinsed and drained
1¼ cups cooked edamame beans
1 tablespoon Easy Hummus
　(see page 92)

Peanut dressing:
1 tablespoon apple cider vinegar
½ teaspoon yellow or grain
　mustard
1 teaspoon honey
1 heaped teaspoon peanut butter
1 tablespoon olive oil
salt and pepper

1. Cook the rice or quinoa in a saucepan of lightly salted boiling water according to packet instructions until tender. Drain.

2. Meanwhile, place all the dressing ingredients in a blender or food processor and blend for 30 seconds, or until smooth.

3. Divide the rice or quinoa, avocado, black beans or chickpeas, edamame beans and hummus between 2 serving bowls and spoon over the dressing. Add your choice of topping.

ENERGIZING SWEET POTATO BUDDHA BOWL

¶¶ serves 2

🎩 10 mins   ⏱ 25 mins

♡ **Buddha Bowl plus topping**

Calories: 765 kcal · Carbohydrates: 68 g · Fat: 39 g · Protein: 27 g

1 tablespoon olive oil
1 teaspoon salt
½ teaspoon black pepper
½ teaspoon chili powder
½ teaspoon paprika
½ teaspoon ground cumin

½ teaspoon garlic powder
  or **1** garlic clove, chopped
2 small sweet potatoes,
  peeled and cut into ½-inch dice
1 quantity Buddha Bowl
  (see opposite)

1. Preheat the oven to 400°F (200°C), and line a baking sheet with parchment paper.

2. Place the olive oil, salt, pepper, spices and garlic in a large bowl and mix well. Add the sweet potatoes and toss to coat thoroughly.

3. Arrange in a single layer on the lined baking sheet and cook for 25 minutes, or until golden, turning halfway through cooking. Serve on top of the Buddha Bowls.

⊕ see overleaf

PROTEIN JALAPEÑO CHICKEN BUDDHA BOWL

 serves 2

🍳 5 mins   ⏱ 10 mins

♡ **Buddha Bowl plus topping**
Calories: 817 kcal · Carbohydrates: 48 g · Fat: 41 g · Protein: 56 g

1 tablespoon olive oil, plus extra for drizzling
1 fresh jalapeño, chopped
1 garlic clove, chopped
1 teaspoon smoked paprika

finely grated zest and juice of **1** lime
2 skinless chicken breasts, sliced
salt
1 quantity Buddha Bowl (see page 110)

1. Place the olive oil, jalapeño, garlic, paprika and lime zest in a bowl. Add most of the lime juice and mix well. Add the chicken, season with salt and toss to coat.

2. Heat a frying pan over medium heat, drizzle in a little olive oil, add the chicken and cook for about 10 minutes until cooked through. Serve on top of your Buddha Bowls, drizzled with the remaining lime juice.

NOURISHING GREENS BUDDHA BOWL

🍴 serves 2

🍳 5 mins   ⏱ 5 mins

♡ **Buddha Bowl plus topping**
Calories: 724 kcal · Carbohydrates: 49 g · Fat: 41 g · Protein: 30 g

1 tablespoon coconut oil
3 garlic cloves, finely chopped
1 fresh jalapeño, chopped
2-inch piece of fresh root ginger, peeled and chopped

1 teaspoon ground turmeric
8 cups kale, spinach or chard (or a mixture), thinly sliced
1 quantity Buddha Bowl (see page 110)

salt
drizzle of lemon juice

1. Heat the coconut oil in a large frying pan over medium heat. Add the garlic, jalapeño, ginger and turmeric and cook for 1 minute.

2. If using kale, remove any thick stalks. Add the greens, stirring thoroughly to coat in the oil, and cook for a few minutes until wilted. Serve on top of your Buddha Bowls, with a sprinkle of salt and a drizzle of lemon juice.

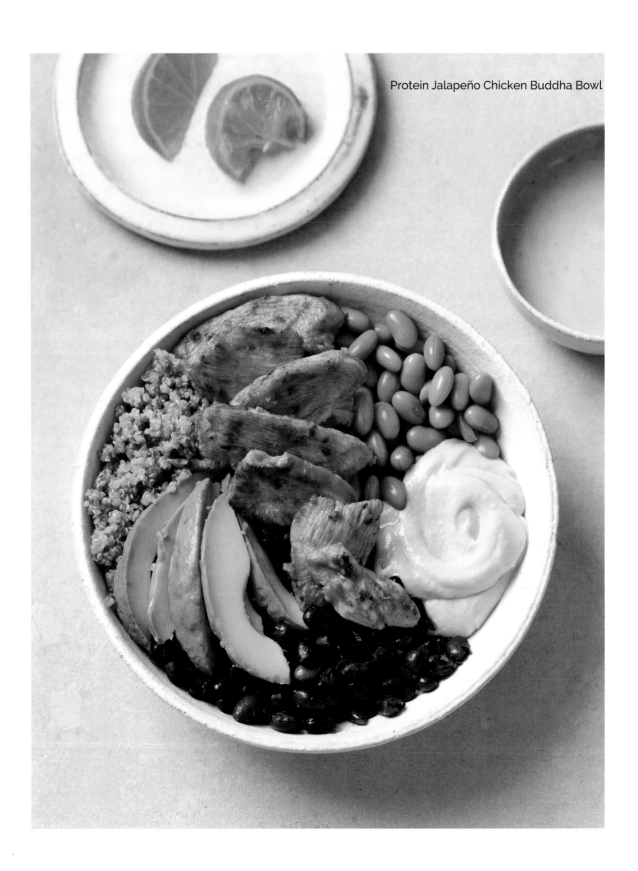

Protein Jalapeño Chicken Buddha Bowl

BYREK

🍴 makes 12 byrek

👨‍🍳 10 mins   ⏱ 30 mins

This is a delicious Albanian recipe, so delicious and so easy to make. The phyllo pastry parcels can be stuffed with a range of different ingredients. I've chosen my favorite here as this is what my mum has always cooked for us, but you could add different vegetables or meat to them too.

Calories: 181 kcal · Carbohydrates: 20 g · Fat: 8.2 g · Protein: 6.5 g

7 cups spinach leaves, finely sliced
2 eggs, beaten
⅔ cup feta cheese, crumbled
2 tablespoons reduced-fat cream
   cheese

salt
12 sheets of phyllo pastry (about 400 g)
4 tablespoons olive oil

---

1. Preheat the oven to 350°F (180°C), and line a baking tray with parchment paper.

2. Place the spinach in a mixing bowl, add the eggs and cheeses, season with salt and mix thoroughly.

3. Lay one sheet of phyllo on a work surface. Place one-twelfth of the spinach mixture along the long edge, leaving a half-inch space between the spinach mixture and the edge of the pastry. Roll the pastry to enclose the filling and make a long

sausage-shaped parcel. Repeat with the remaining ingredients to make 12 parcels.

4. Curve the *byrek* into horseshoe shapes and arrange on the lined baking sheet. Brush olive oil all over the byrek and sprinkle with a little salt. Cook for 30 minutes, or until golden.

5. Any leftovers can be stored in an airtight container in the refrigerator for up to 3 days.

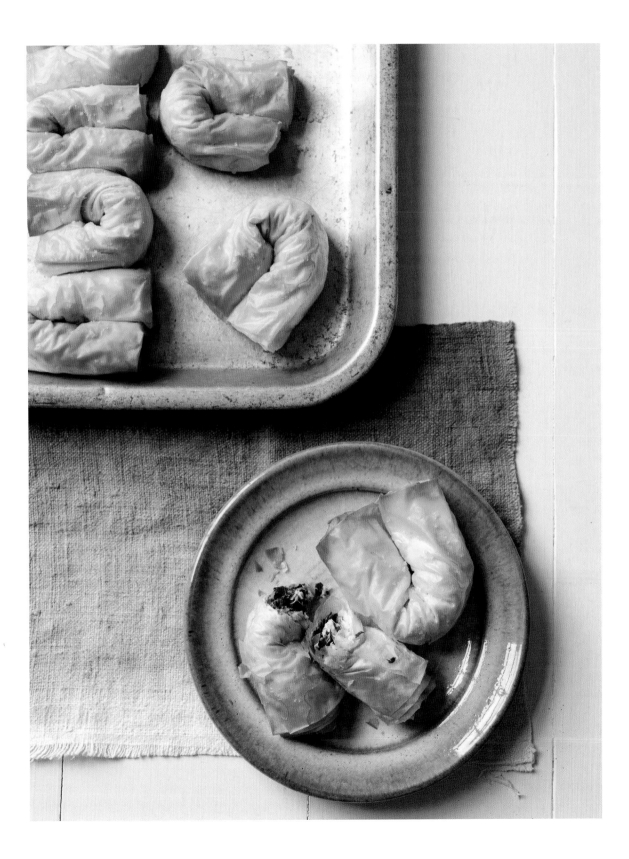

PAN-FRIED SALMON WITH COCONUT GREENS

¶¶ serves 2, generously

🎩 10 mins   ⏱ 15 mins

I love this super-quick meal as a tasty lunch or a lovely dinner. I really like salmon, and so many of my clients love eating it too. You can add any veg you like—just see what you've got in the refrigerator and throw it in!

Calories: 360 kcal • Carbohydrates: 5.5 g • Fat: 26.6 g • Protein: 27.4 g

1 tablespoon olive oil
2 salmon fillets with skin
salt
8 cups greens (such as kale, spinach or cavolo nero), thinly sliced

1 tablespoon coconut oil
¾-inch piece of fresh root ginger, peeled and chopped
3 garlic cloves, finely chopped
juice of **1** lemon

1. Heat the olive oil in a frying pan over medium heat. Sprinkle the salmon skin with salt, then cook skin side down for about 8 minutes until the skin is crisp and the salmon is nearly cooked through. Turn the fillets and cook for 1 minute on the other side. Remove from the pan and keep warm.

2. Meanwhile, if using kale, remove the thick stalks.

3. Add the coconut oil to the salmon pan and melt. Add the ginger and garlic and then the greens, stir and cook for a few minutes until the greens have wilted. Squeeze over the lemon juice and season with salt. Divide between 2 plates and top with the salmon fillets.

VEGGIE NOODLES WITH WALNUT PESTO

🍴 serves 4

👨‍🍳 10 mins   ⏱ 5 mins

This is super easy and super quick—perfect for a busy day! I love using zucchini or butternut squash noodles to get my vegetables in. Of course, you could use egg or rice noodles instead, but veggie noodles add a nice bit of flavor and extra nutrition.

Calories: 471 kcal · Carbohydrates: 10 g · Fat: 41 g · Protein: 14 g

Walnut pesto:
4 cups basil leaves
1½ cups walnuts
2 garlic cloves, peeled
½ cup grated Parmesan cheese, plus extra to serve
3 tablespoons extra-virgin olive oil
3–4 tablespoons water

salt and pepper
olive oil, for frying
4 cups veggie noodles, such as zucchini or butternut squash

1. To make the walnut pesto, place the basil, walnuts, garlic and Parmesan in a blender or food processor and blend to a thick paste, scraping the sides as you go. Add the extra-virgin olive oil and the measured water, 1 tablespoon at a time, and keep blending until you have a smooth paste. Season with salt and pepper to taste.

2. Heat the olive oil in a large saucepan and cook the noodles for about 1 minute until warmed through. Add the pesto to the pan and stir well until mixed. Serve with a little extra Parmesan.

✍ TIP
For extra protein, top each serving of noodles with 1 cooked and sliced chicken breast or 1 cooked salmon fillet.

↪ SWAP
Vegan *Swap the Parmesan for 2 tablespoons of nutritional yeast.*

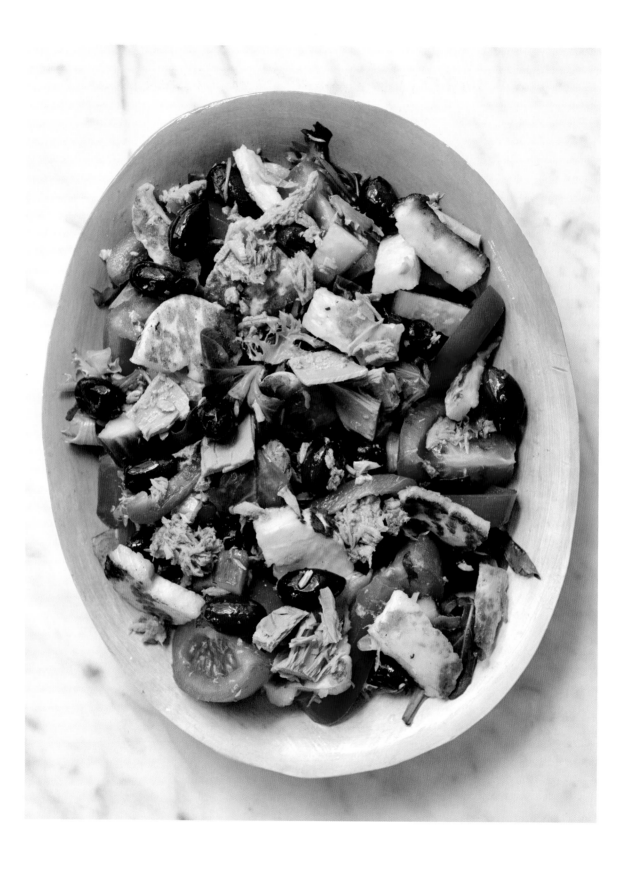

MEDITERRANEAN TUNA WITH HALLOUMI

¶¶ serves 2, generously

♨ 10 mins   **⏱ 5 mins**

This delicious, protein-filled salad is perfect for lunch or even dinner on a hot day. I absolutely love the flavor of black olives with Halloumi, and this salad takes next to no time to put together. It is ideal for packed lunches or meal prep as it can be kept in the refrigerator for a couple of days.

Calories: 735 kcal · Carbohydrates: 33.2 g · Fat: 47.2 g · Protein: 51.2 g

8 ounces Halloumi cheese, thickly sliced
1–2 tablespoons olive oil, plus extra for frying
4 large tomatoes, cut into wedges
1 cucumber, diced

1 pepper, cored, deseeded and sliced
½ cup pitted black olives
juice of **1** lemon
7 cups salad leaves (I like arugula)
5-ounce can tuna in water, drained
salt and pepper

1. Pat the Halloumi with a paper towel to dry off the moisture. Heat a drizzle of the olive oil in a frying pan over medium-high heat, add the Halloumi and cook for about 2 minutes on each side until golden brown.

2. Place all the remaining ingredients in a large serving bowl and season well with salt and pepper. Add the Halloumi and toss everything to coat in the olive oil and lemon juice, then serve.

⤶ SWAP

Vegan Swap the Halloumi for firm tofu and cook in the same way. Swap the tuna for a can of chickpeas, rinsed and drained.

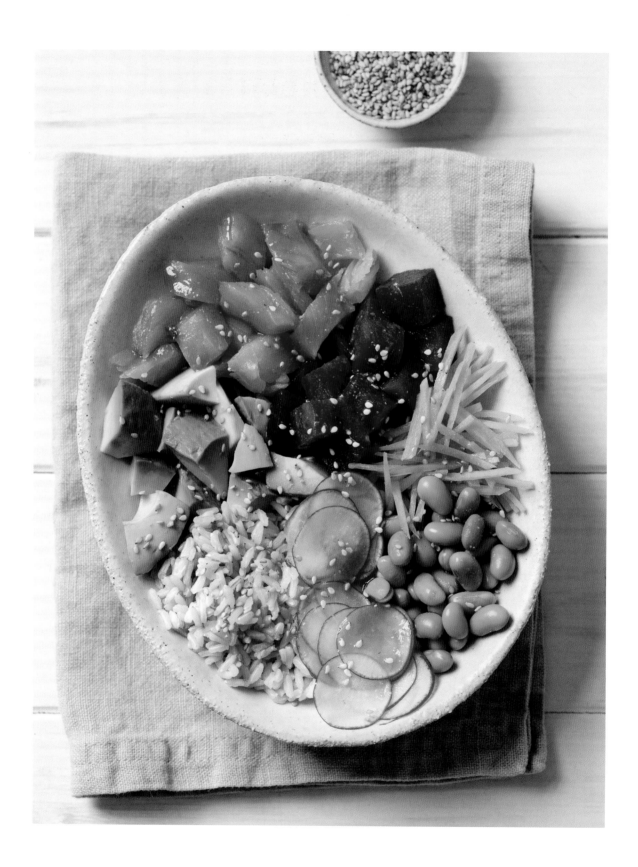

POKE BOWL

¶¶ serves 2, generously
♨ 15 mins, plus cooling and marinating   **⏱ 25 mins**

I love making myself a poke bowl to take to work. It's so quick and easy to put together, and I love all the different types of veggies I can add to it. I wouldn't usually eat radish and beets on their own, so this is a great way to add them into my diet. This is perfect for me and now for you too!

Calories: 660 kcal · Carbohydrates: 48 g · Fat: 33 g · Protein: 36 g

⅓ cup brown rice

Marinade:
1 tablespoon tamari
1 tablespoon honey or
   maple syrup
½ tablespoon sesame oil

1 teaspoon miso paste
juice of **1** lime

1 cooked beet, diced
7 ounces smoked salmon
¾ cup cooked edamame
   beans

handful of radishes, sliced
2 carrots, peeled and cut
   into strips
1 avocado, cubed
sesame seeds, for
   sprinkling

1. Cook the rice in a saucepan of lightly salted boiling water according to packet instructions until tender. Drain and allow to cool.

2. Mix all the marinade ingredients in a bowl, add the beet and stir to coat. Leave to marinate for 10 minutes, then drain, reserving the marinade.

3. To assemble the poke bowls, start by placing the rice to one side. Then arrange all the ingredients around it as you wish, getting creative and making your poke bowl beautiful. Finish with a sprinkling of sesame seeds, then drizzle the reserved marinade over the top.

⤷ SWAP
Vegan Swap the smoked salmon for 1 cup of diced watermelon.

THE BEST TUNA PASTA SALAD

🍴 serves 2, generously

👨‍🍳 10 mins, plus cooling   ⏱ 15 mins

I love Italian food, so adding pasta to my salad is always going to work for me. This is a really tasty and balanced lunch and one you might usually pick up in the supermarket, am I right? Well, now you can make it as you meal prep and keep a couple of portions in the refrigerator to save you time during the week. This is a great meal to take to work and look forward to at lunchtime—enjoy!

Calories: 708 kcal · Carbohydrates: 71 g · Fat: 20 g · Protein: 54 g

1½ cups whole wheat pasta (I like using *casarecce*)

Dressing:
120 ml plain yogurt
1 tablespoon yellow or grain mustard
juice of **1** lemon

1 tablespoon apple cider vinegar
salt and pepper

2 x 5-ounce cans tuna in brine, drained and flaked
8-ounce can sweet corn, drained

½ cup pitted black olives, halved
2 hard-boiled eggs, chopped
1 red onion, finely chopped
2 celery sticks, chopped
handful of chopped parsley, to garnish

1. Cook the pasta in a saucepan of lightly salted boiling water according to packet instructions until tender. Drain and allow to cool.

2. Place all the dressing ingredients in a small bowl and whisk to combine. Season with salt and pepper to taste.

3. Place all the remaining salad ingredients in a large serving bowl with the pasta, pour over the dressing and mix well. Garnish with chopped parsley.

⤷SWAP

Vegan Swap the tuna for a can of chickpeas or kidney beans, rinsed and drained. Swap the eggs for a handful of walnuts and use vegan yogurt.

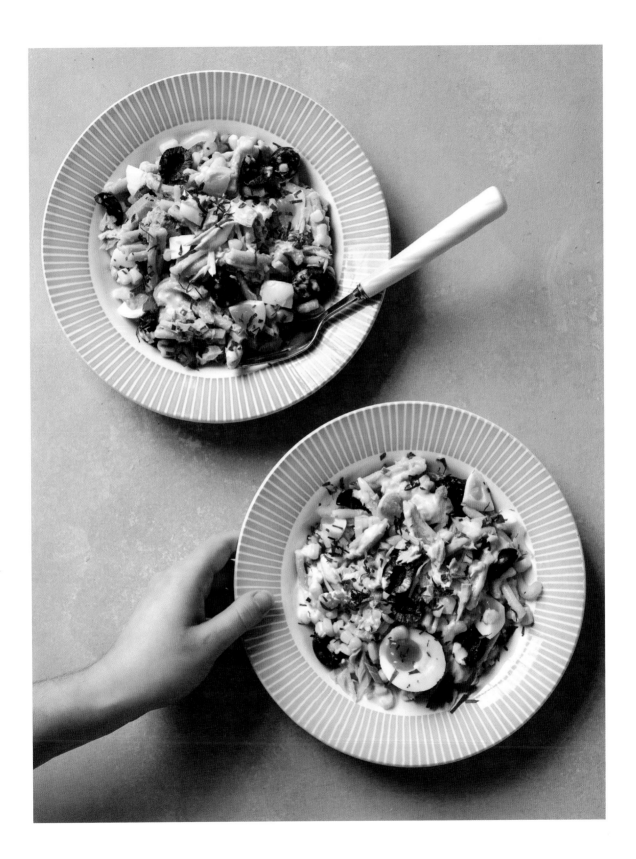

RAMEN THREE WAYS

🍴 serves 2

👨‍🍳 10 mins   ⏱ 15 mins

Another versatile, colorful and delicious meal that gets you excited for lunch!
Food doesn't need to be dull—it can be creative, nourishing and offer the
perfect amount of fuel. Ramen isn't just something you get at a restaurant—you
can make your own using so many different ingredients. Thai Coconut Shrimp
(see page 127) is my absolute go-to. Follow the recipe to make the basic ramen,
then choose one of the toppings to complete your bowl.

Calories: 142 kcal · Carbohydrates: 17.2 g · Fat: 6.1 g · Protein: 5 g

2 tablespoons miso paste
handful of dried seaweed
  (optional)
handful of dried shiitake
  mushrooms or fresh
  white mushrooms
4 cups water
1 slice of fresh root ginger

1 tablespoon tamari
¾ cup dried noodles
2 handfuls of raw chopped
  veggies (such as bok choi,
  bean sprouts, spinach, thinly
  sliced carrot or radish)
1 fresh jalapeño, sliced (optional)

1. Place the miso paste, seaweed (if using),
mushrooms and measured water in a saucepan
over high heat and bring to a boil. Add the ginger
and tamari, reduce the heat and simmer
for 10 minutes.

2. Meanwhile, cook the noodles in a saucepan of
lightly salted boiling water according to packet
instructions until tender. Drain and divide between
2 large bowls. Arrange the raw veggies on top.

3. Strain the hot miso broth through a sieve into the
bowls. Add the sliced jalapeño, if using, and your
choice of topping.

📝 TIP

*After straining the hot broth into my bowl, I like
to slice the mushrooms and seaweed and add
them to the ramen with my choice of topping.*

CHICKEN & GINGER RAMEN

¶¶ serves 2

👒 10 mins　　　　⏱ 10 mins

♡ **Ramen plus topping**
Calories: 382 kcal · Carbohydrates: 37.2 g · Fat: 20.1 g · Protein: 14.7 g

finely grated zest and juice
　of **1** orange
1 tablespoon honey
2 tablespoons soy sauce
2 tablespoons rice vinegar

1 tablespoon sesame oil
¾-inch piece of fresh root
　ginger, finely grated, or
　½ teaspoon ground ginger
pinch of crushed red pepper

2 skinless chicken breasts,
　sliced
olive oil, for frying
1 quantity Ramen (see
　opposite)

1. Place all the ingredients, except the chicken, olive oil and ramen, in a bowl and mix well. Add the sliced chicken and toss to coat.

2. Heat a frying pan over medium heat, drizzle in a little olive oil, add the chicken and cook, stirring, for about 10 minutes until tender and cooked through. Serve on top of the ramen.

TOFU SATAY RAMEN

¶¶ serves 2

👒 5 mins　　　　⏱ 15 mins

♡ **Ramen plus topping**
Calories: 383 kcal · Carbohydrates: 29.9 g · Fat: 21.3 g · Protein: 23.7 g

juice of **1** lime
1 teaspoon honey
1 tablespoon soy sauce

1 tablespoon curry powder
3 tablespoons smooth peanut
　butter

1 cup firm tofu, sliced
1 quantity Ramen (see
　opposite)

1. Preheat the oven to 350°F (180°C), and line a baking sheet with parchment paper.

2. Mix all the ingredients, except the tofu and ramen, in a bowl until smooth.

3. Dip the tofu in the mixture, then arrange on the lined baking sheet. Cook for 15 minutes, turning once, or until golden. Serve on top of the ramen.

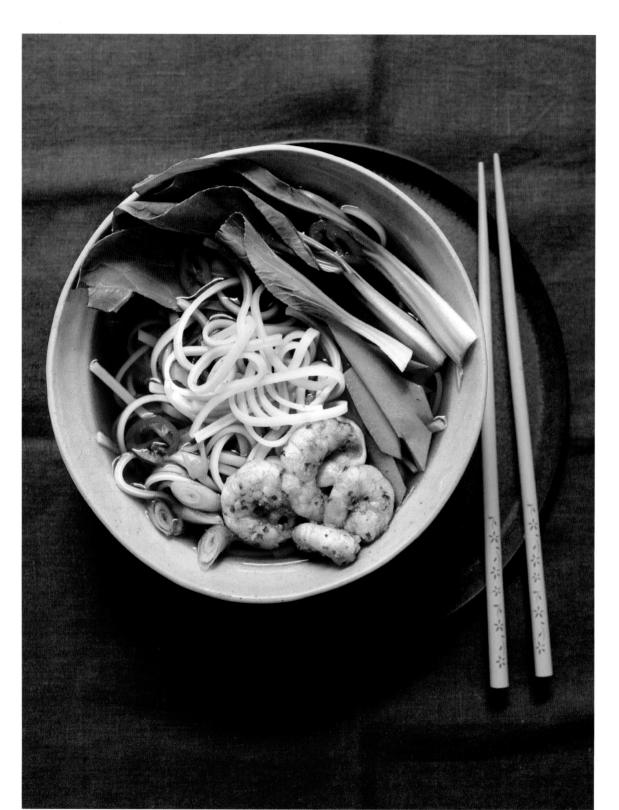

THAI COCONUT SHRIMP RAMEN

¶¶ serves 2

👨‍🍳 **10 mins**   ⏱ **5 mins**

♡ **Ramen plus topping**

Calories: 518 kcal · Carbohydrates: 30.4 g · Fat: 38.5 g · Protein: 18.4 g

---

¾-inch piece of fresh root ginger, finely grated, or **½ teaspoon** ground ginger

1 lemongrass stalk, tough outer leaves removed

2 garlic cloves, peeled

1 jalapeño, stalk removed

finely grated zest and juice of **1** lime

2 tablespoons soy sauce

3.5 ounces creamed coconut, chopped

12 large shrimp

drizzle of coconut oil

1 quantity Ramen (see page 124)

1. Place all the ingredients, except the shrimp, coconut oil and ramen, in a blender or food processor and blend to a thick, rough paste. Transfer to a bowl and add the shrimp. Mix until well coated.

2. Heat a drizzle of coconut oil in a frying pan over high heat and add the shrimp. Cook for 2–3 minutes until pink and just cooked through. Serve on top of the ramen.

SUPER GREEN CAESAR SALAD

🍴 serves 2, generously

🍳 15 mins　　　　　⏱ 20 mins

You can get creative with this recipe, adding the veggies you fancy or those you have left in your refrigerator. That's the best thing about a salad: you can toss almost anything in, and it will taste lovely.

Calories: 824 kcal · Carbohydrates: 28 g · Fat: 48 g · Protein: 65 g

2 garlic cloves, finely chopped
2 tablespoons olive oil, plus extra for drizzling
juice of **1** lemon
salt and pepper
2 skinless chicken breasts, each sliced into 4 pieces
2 slices of stale whole-grain bread, cut into chunks

3 cups kale, stalks removed, chopped
Dressing:
1 cup plain yogurt
1 tablespoon olive oil
2 garlic cloves, crushed
4 canned anchovy fillets, finely chopped
juice of **1** lemon

3 tablespoons grated Parmesan cheese
2 hard-boiled eggs, cut into wedges
½ avocado, sliced
handful of chopped parsley
1 tablespoon Parmesan cheese shavings

1. Preheat the oven to 350°F (180°C), and line a baking sheet with parchment paper.

2. Place the chopped garlic in a small bowl with 1 tablespoon of the olive oil and the lemon juice and season well with salt and pepper. Dip the chunks of chicken in the mixture and place on the lined baking sheet. Cook for 20 minutes, or until tender and cooked through.

3. Meanwhile, spread the bread chunks on another baking sheet. Drizzle with the remaining olive oil and a sprinkle of salt. Toss to coat and cook for 10 minutes, until golden and crispy. These are the croutons.

4. Place the kale in a large serving bowl. Sprinkle with ½ teaspoon of salt and drizzle with a little olive oil. Use your hands to massage the kale for 2–3 minutes to soften it.

5. Place all the dressing ingredients in a small bowl and whisk to combine. Season to taste.

6. Place the cooked chicken, eggs, avocado and croutons in the bowl with the kale. Pour the dressing over and mix thoroughly. Sprinkle with the parsley and Parmesan shavings.

⤷SWAP

Vegan Swap the Parmesan for nutritional yeast, swap the chicken for 1 can of chickpeas, rinsed and drained, and swap the anchovy fillets for 1 tablespoon of capers.

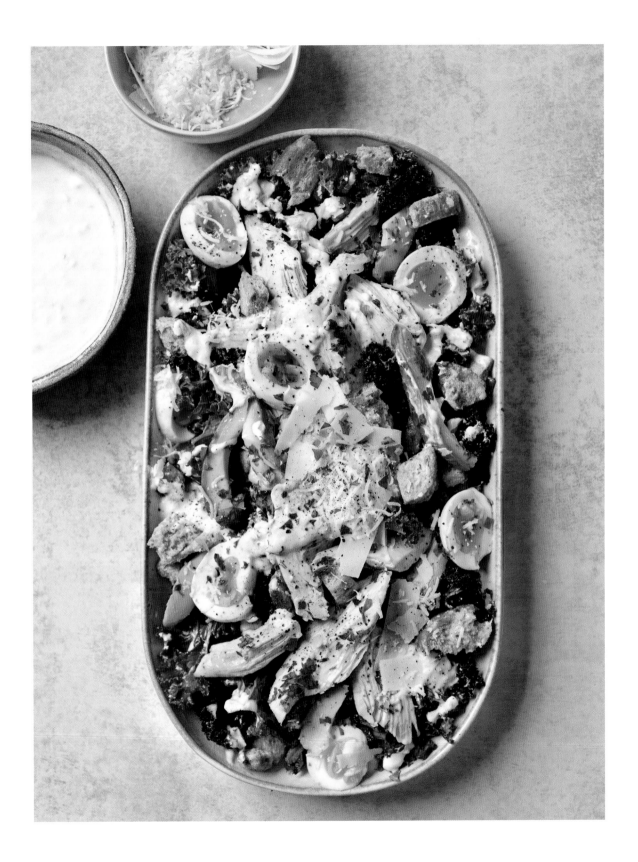

TURKISH PIZZA

serves 2

15 mins · 15 mins

Turkish pizza makes such a nice change from traditional Italian pizza. I love snacking on flatbread, and now I can have flatbread with all my favorite pizza toppings—that's food heaven for me! Sumac is such a lovely Middle Eastern spice, adding a gorgeous flavor. This is a great one for lunch with friends.

Calories: 488 kcal · Carbohydrates: 24 g · Fat: 35 g · Protein: 18 g

2 whole wheat flatbreads

Topping:
1 small onion, peeled and quartered
2 garlic cloves, peeled
1 large tomato
1 tablespoon harissa paste

handful of parsley leaves
1 teaspoon ground cinnamon
1 teaspoon grated nutmeg
1 teaspoon dried thyme
5 ounces lean ground lamb
2 teaspoons sumac

Additional toppings:
handful of mint leaves
1 red onion, sliced

Optional extras:
chopped fresh tomatoes, crumbled feta cheese, sliced jalapeños

1. Preheat the oven to 400°F (200°C), and place the flatbreads on a baking sheet.

2. Place all the topping ingredients in a blender or food processor and blend to a paste.

3. Spread the topping in an even layer over the flatbreads, pressing it down so it sticks to the dough. Cook for 10–15 minutes until golden and sizzling.

4. Top the pizzas with the mint leaves, red onion and any of the optional extras you fancy. Serve flat or roll up as a wrap.

⤷ SWAP
Vegan Swap the meat for vegan mince or 2 cups of chopped walnuts.

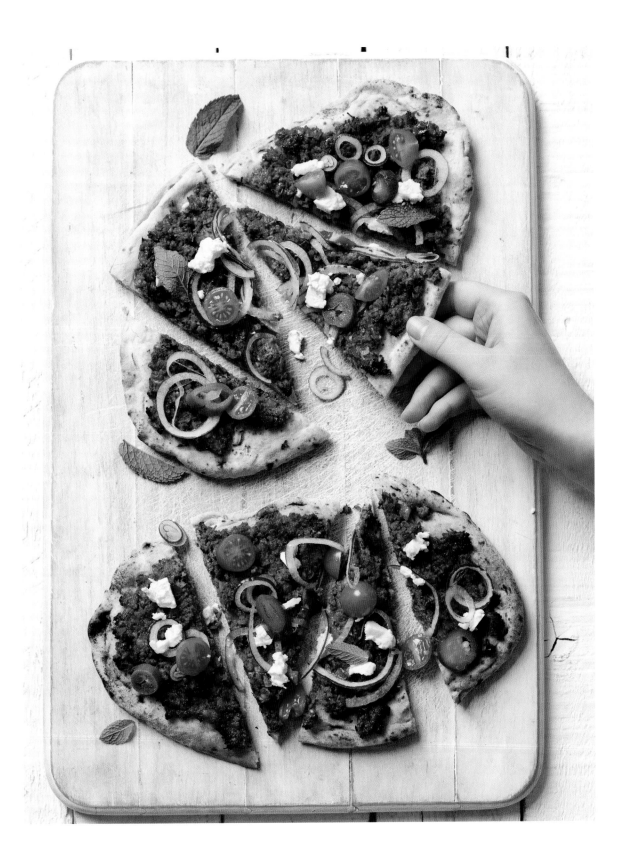

DINNER

THREE-BEAN CHILI BOWL

serves 4

10 mins   **30 mins**

Who doesn't love Mexican food? I love chili—it's so comforting, nourishing and a great option for batch cooking. I usually cook up a batch and keep it in the refrigerator or freezer in portions. Then all I need to do is boil a bit of rice every time I fancy it—easy! This is one of my favorite vegetarian recipes, full of protein and so much flavor.

Calories: 675 kcal · Carbohydrates: 100 g · Fat: 20 g · Protein: 28 g

2 tablespoons olive oil
1 large onion, chopped
1 garlic clove, crushed
1 teaspoon ground cumin
1 teaspoon ground cinnamon
1 teaspoon ground coriander
1 teaspoon smoked paprika
1 teaspoon chili powder

15-ounce can kidney beans, rinsed and drained
15-ounce can chickpeas, rinsed and drained
15-ounce can butter beans, rinsed and drained
2 x 14.5-ounce cans diced tomatoes
juice of **2** limes

½ cup water
salt and pepper

Serving suggestions:
brown rice
sour cream or plain yogurt
sliced avocado
sliced fresh jalapeño

1. Heat the olive oil in a large saucepan over medium-low heat, add the onion and garlic and cook for about 5 minutes until softened. Stir in the spices and cook for a further 2 minutes. Add all the remaining ingredients, season well with salt and pepper and simmer for about 20 minutes until thickened and reduced.

2. Serve the chili in bowls on a bed of rice, topped with a spoonful of sour cream or yogurt and the sliced avocado. Sprinkle the sliced fresh jalapeño over the top.

✎ TIP

Leftover chili is delicious eaten cold in a wrap with some salad leaves for lunch. Alternatively, place the chili in an ovenproof dish, top with a layer of mashed sweet potato and bake for 30 minutes at 350˚F (180˚C), for a Chili Shepherd's Pie.

PASTA THREE WAYS

Pasta is super quick, super easy and super tasty too! You can get creative with your pasta sauces and add all the veggies and spices you enjoy to make your own personal sauce. I've shared my favorite pasta sauce recipes here. I hope you love them as much as I do. I serve the sauces with pasta, but you can serve them with vegetable noodles, such as zucchini or butternut noodles.

CHICKEN ALFREDO

🍴 serves 2

👨‍🍳 5 mins   ⏱ 10 mins

Calories: 535 kcal · Carbohydrates: 28 g · Fat: 22 g · Protein: 54 g

1½ cups pasta (I like tagliatelle)
1 tablespoon olive oil
1 garlic clove, chopped
½ cup Greek yogurt

½ cup grated Parmesan cheese, plus extra for sprinkling
a little white wine or water (optional)
2 cooked chicken fillets, sliced
salt and pepper

1. Cook the pasta in a saucepan of lightly salted boiling water according to packet instructions until tender. Drain and return to the pan.

2. Meanwhile, heat the olive oil in a saucepan over low heat. Add the garlic and cook for 1 minute, stirring, then add the yogurt and Parmesan and whisk until smooth. If the sauce is too thick, add a little white wine or water to thin it. Add the chicken to the pan and cook for 2 minutes until the chicken is piping hot, then season with salt and pepper to taste.

3. Stir the sauce through the pasta and serve with an extra sprinkling of Parmesan.

⤷ SWAP

Vegan Blend the flesh from 2 avocados with ½ cup of milk of your choice, 1 tablespoon of nutritional yeast and 1 teaspoon of ground cashews. Cook the garlic in the oil as above, then stir in the avocado mixture, season to taste and cook for 2 minutes.

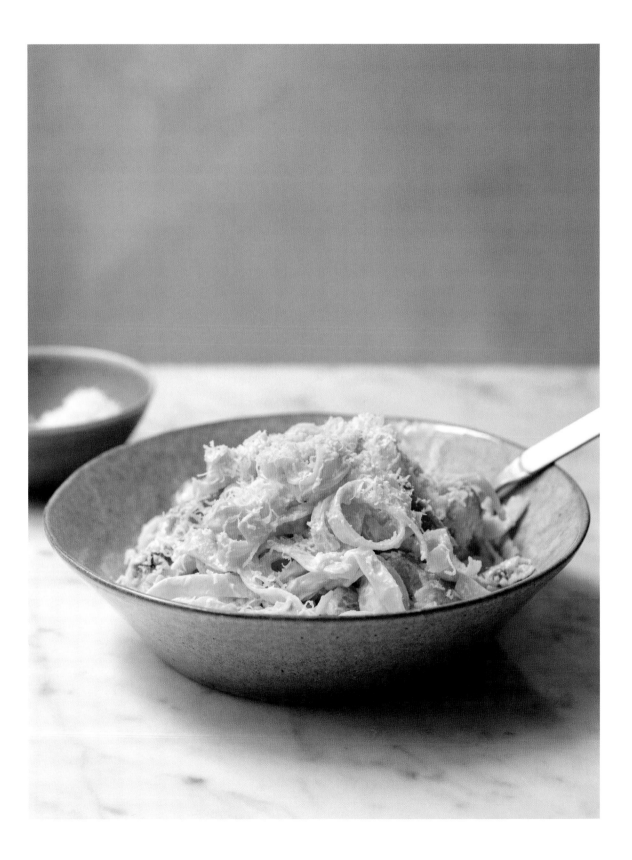

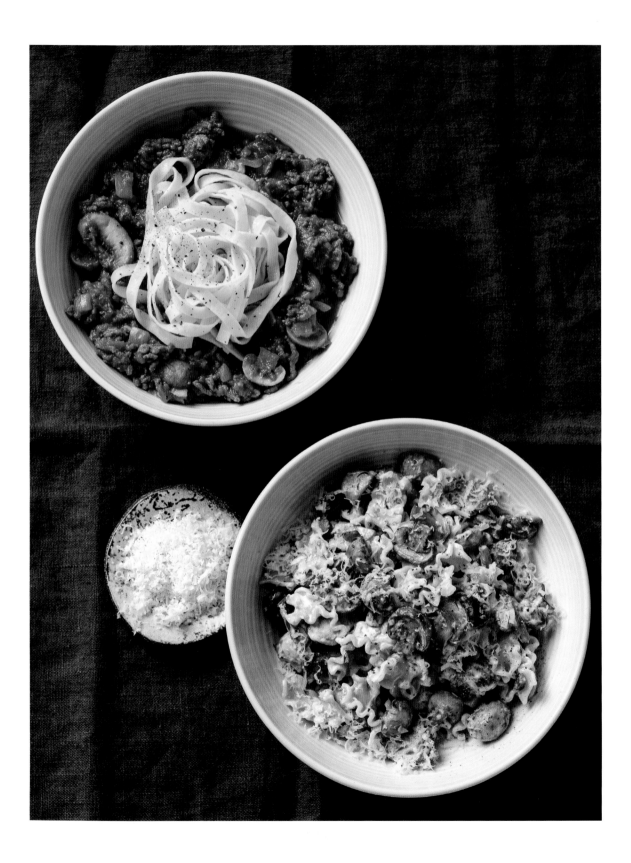

PASTA BOLOGNESE

serves 2

10 mins ⏱ 10 mins

Calories: 892 kcal · Carbohydrates: 81 g · Fat: 30 g · Protein: 67 g

2 cups pasta (I like tagliatelle)
½ quantity of Bolognese Sauce (see page 158)
grated Parmesan cheese, to serve

1. Cook the pasta in a saucepan of lightly salted boiling water according to packet instructions until tender. Drain and return to the pan.

2. Meanwhile, place the Bolognese sauce in a saucepan and cook for a few minutes until piping hot.

3. Stir the sauce through the pasta and serve with a sprinkling of Parmesan.

GARLIC MUSHROOM PASTA

serves 2

5 mins ⏱ 10 mins

Calories: 694 kcal · Carbohydrates: 37 g · Fat: 37 g · Protein: 24 g

180 g pasta (I like whole wheat Mafalda *corta*)
2 tablespoons olive oil
2 cups mushrooms, chopped or sliced
2 garlic cloves, chopped
1 teaspoon fresh or dried thyme

finely grated zest and juice of **1** lemon
salt and pepper
2 tablespoons crème fraîche
½ cup grated Parmesan cheese, plus extra to serve

1. Cook the pasta in a saucepan of lightly salted boiling water according to packet instructions until tender. Drain and return to the pan.

2. Meanwhile, heat the olive oil in a large saucepan over medium heat. Add the mushrooms and cook for about 5 minutes until browned, stirring occasionally. Add the garlic, thyme and lemon zest and season well with salt and pepper. Cook for about 2 minutes, stirring, then add the crème fraîche, Parmesan and lemon juice and stir in.

3. Stir the sauce through the pasta and serve with an extra sprinkling of Parmesan.

RICOTTA & SPINACH PASTA

¶¶ serves 3, generously

🍳 15 mins, plus cooling   ⏱ 55 mins

Pasta just keeps getting better and better! If I have a bit more time in the kitchen and really fancy a little something extra, I pick up some cannelloni or large pasta shells and make this super-yummy meal.

Calories: 417 kcal · Carbohydrates: 31.3 g · Fat: 28 g · Protein: 14 g

16 cannelloni or large pasta shells

Tomato sauce:
3 tablespoons olive oil
1 large onion, chopped
2 garlic cloves, crushed
2 x 14.5-ounce cans diced tomatoes

1 tablespoon tomato purée
1 teaspoon dried basil
1 teaspoon dried oregano
1 teaspoon sugar

1 tablespoon olive oil
2 garlic cloves, chopped

7 cups spinach leaves, roughly chopped
¼ cup mozzarella cheese, grated, plus extra for sprinkling
⅔ cup ricotta cheese
6 basil leaves, finely chopped
salt and pepper

1. Preheat the oven to 350°F (180°C).

2. Cook the cannelloni or pasta shells in a large saucepan of lightly salted boiling water according to packet instructions, then drain and allow to cool.

3. For the tomato sauce, heat the olive oil in a large saucepan over medium-low heat, add the onion and garlic and cook for about 5 minutes until softened. Add the remaining sauce ingredients and bring to a boil, then lower the heat and simmer for 15 minutes. Season with salt and pepper to taste.

4. Meanwhile, heat the tablespoon of olive oil in a frying pan over medium heat, add the garlic and cook for 1 minute, stirring. Add the spinach and cook for about 3 minutes until wilted. Transfer the spinach to a large

bowl, add the mozzarella, ricotta and basil, season thoroughly with salt and pepper and mix to combine.

5. Spread half the tomato sauce over the base of an ovenproof dish in which the cannelloni or pasta shells fit snugly in one layer. Stuff the pasta with a generous amount of the spinach mixture and arrange in the ovenproof dish. Top with the rest of the tomato sauce, sprinkle over a little grated mozzarella, cover the dish with foil and cook for 15 minutes. Remove the foil and cook for another 10 minutes, until bubbling.

⤷SWAP

Vegan Swap the ricotta for vegan cream cheese and the mozzarella for 1 tablespoon of nutritional yeast.

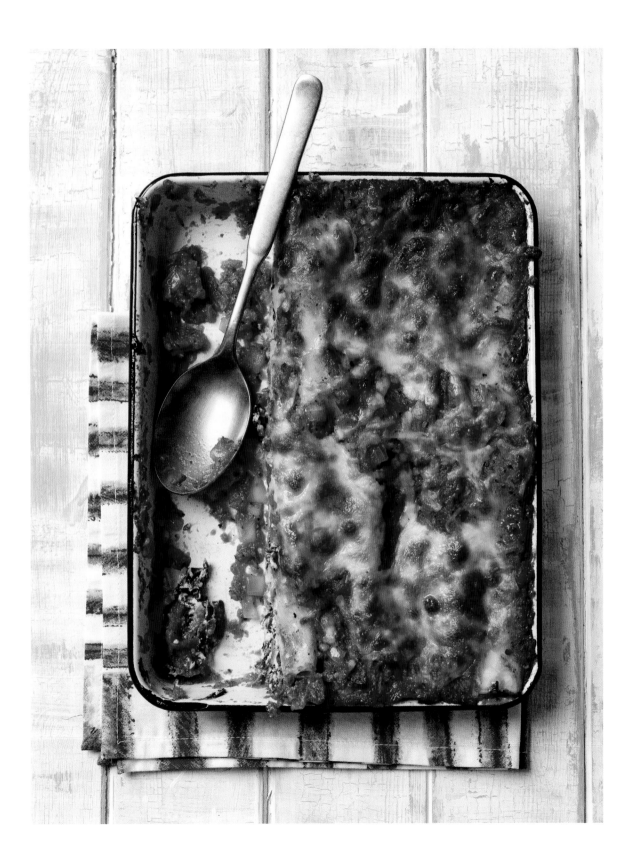

BURANI

¶¶ serves 2

⌂ **10 mins**   ⏱ **25 mins**

I love my mumma's cooking, and this is one of my favorite Albanian dishes, so I had to share the recipe with you! When my mum makes this, I can eat it for breakfast, lunch and dinner. Have it hot or cold, it is so delicious. I can't wait for you to try it. *Ju bëftë mirë!*

Calories: 441 kcal · Carbohydrates: 36 g · Fat: 23 g · Protein: 20 g

1 tablespoon butter
1 tablespoon olive oil
1 onion, chopped
⅓ cup long-grain rice

1 liter boiling water
7 cups spinach leaves
salt and pepper
4 eggs

a few torn basil leaves, to garnish

---

1. Heat the butter and olive oil in a large saucepan over medium heat, add the onion and cook for a few minutes to soften. Add the rice and stir continuously for 1 minute, then add the boiling water, taking care as it will spit. Cover with a lid, bring to a boil and cook for 10 minutes.

2. Add the spinach and stir until it wilts. Bring the mixture back to a boil and cook for about 5 minutes, uncovered, until there is only a small amount of liquid left at the bottom of the pan. Season thoroughly with salt and pepper.

3. Crack the eggs over the top of the *burani*, cover with a lid and cook for 3–4 minutes until the egg whites are set. Watch carefully as you do not want to overcook the eggs. Remove the pan from the heat and leave to stand for 5 minutes before serving with the torn basil sprinkled on top.

⤷**SWAP**

Vegan Replace the eggs with some diced, firm tofu.

☑**TIP**

Any leftovers are delicious cold the next day made into a salad. Stir in 1 can of tuna, drained, 1 small can of sweet corn, drained, 1 chopped red pepper and some chopped parsley.

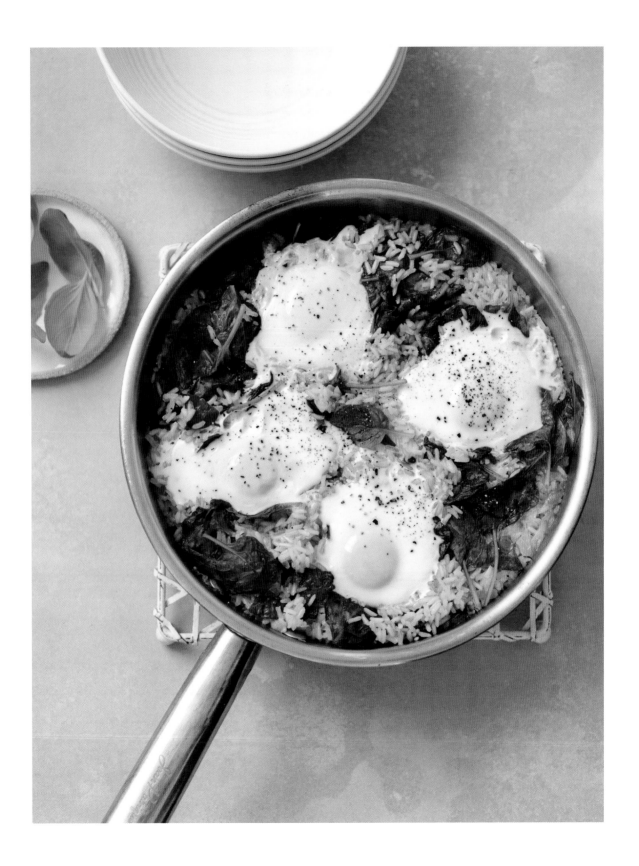

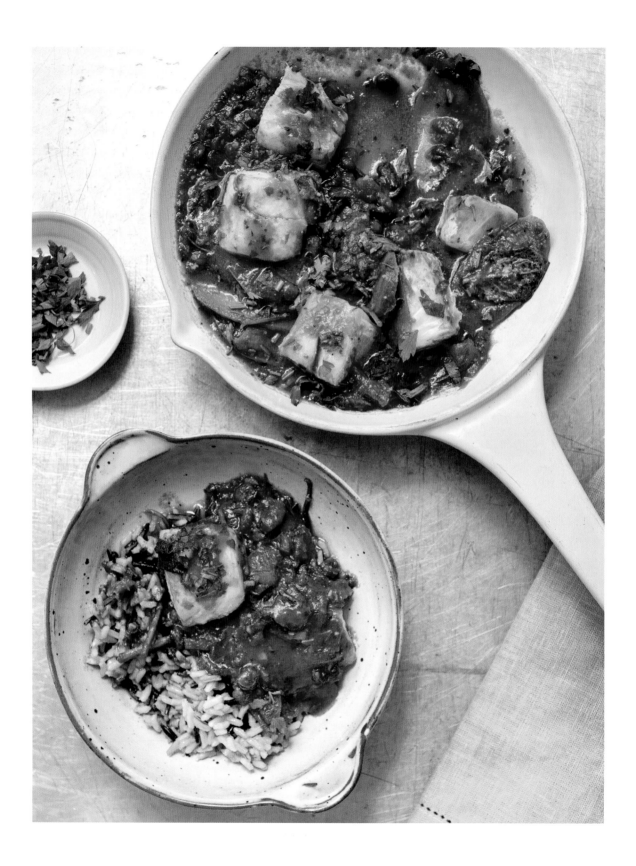

SPANISH STEW WITH COD

🍴 serves 2, generously

👨‍🍳 10 mins **⏱ 30 mins**

Baked cod is so tasty, and this recipe makes me hungry just thinking about it—it's something you might enjoy in a lovely, cozy restaurant, but now you can make it in your very own kitchen. There is quite a bit to it, but it makes a great Friday dinner or a meal for when you have company. It's rich in protein, making it perfect after a workout.

> Calories: 408 kcal · Carbohydrates: 49.9 g · Fat: 10.4 g · Protein: 32.2 g

1 tablespoon olive oil
1 onion, sliced
1 leek, sliced
2 garlic cloves, chopped
1-inch piece of fresh root ginger, peeled and chopped
pinch of ground cayenne
pinch of smoked paprika

3 carrots, scrubbed and sliced
14.5-ounce can diced tomatoes
1 teaspoon honey or maple syrup
2¼ cups vegetable stock
1 tablespoon soy sauce
5 cups spinach leaves

⅓ cup capers, drained
handful of roughly chopped parsley
salt and pepper
2 cod fillets, cut into chunks

Serving suggestion:
cooked wild rice

1. Heat the olive oil in a large saucepan over medium heat. Add the onion and leek and fry for 2–3 minutes, then add the garlic, ginger, cayenne, paprika and carrots. Fry for 2 minutes before adding the tomatoes, honey or maple syrup, stock and soy sauce. Bring to a simmer and cook for 5 minutes.

2. Stir in the spinach and capers, then simmer for a further 10 minutes. Add the parsley and season with salt and pepper to taste.

3. Meanwhile, preheat the oven to 400°F (200°C), and lightly grease a baking sheet. Arrange the cod on the baking sheet. Season well with salt and pepper and cook for about 10 minutes until golden and almost cooked through.

4. Stir the cod into the stew and cook for a further 5 minutes. Serve in bowls on a bed of wild rice.

FISH PIE OF DREAMS

⚔ serves 4

👨‍🍳 **15 mins**   ⏱ **1 hour**

When you can't decide what fish to have for dinner, eat them all in my fish pie of dreams! So warm, nourishing and satisfying, this is a great dinner for the family or just before a movie night—it leaves your tummy feeling very, very happy. Any leftovers can be frozen in portions for a quick-and-tasty ready meal.

Calories: 595 kcal · Carbohydrates: 17 g · Fat: 43 g · Protein: 38 g

Cauliflower mash:
1 large cauliflower, cut into small florets
1 tablespoon olive oil
1 tablespoon crème fraîche
pinch of grated nutmeg
salt and pepper

2 skinless salmon fillets, cut into chunks

2 skinless white fish fillets, cut into chunks
2 skinless mackerel fillets, cut into chunks
¾ cup crème fraîche
½ cup water
1 red onion, finely chopped
2 bay leaves
a few cloves
pinch of grated nutmeg

1 teaspoon yellow or grain mustard
¾ cup Cheddar cheese, grated
juice of **1** lemon
4 hard-boiled eggs, quartered
4 tablespoons snipped chives

1. First make the cauliflower mash. Cook the cauliflower in a large saucepan of lightly salted water for about 10 minutes until tender, then drain well. Transfer to a blender or food processor with the olive oil, crème fraîche and nutmeg, season well with salt and pepper and blend until smooth and creamy. Set aside.

2. Preheat the oven to 400°F (200°C). Place the fish in a deep saucepan and pour in the crème fraîche and measured water. Add the onion, bay leaves and cloves to the pan and season well. Place the pan over medium heat and bring to a simmer, then reduce the heat and cook for about 5 minutes until the fish is cooked through.

3. Use a slotted spoon to transfer the fish to a shallow ovenproof dish and set aside. Add the nutmeg and mustard to the sauce in the pan and simmer over gentle heat for about 5 minutes until it starts to thicken. Discard the bay leaves and cloves. Add ½ cup of the cheese and the lemon juice and stir until melted and thickened. Season to taste with salt and pepper.

4. Place the egg quarters in the ovenproof dish on top of the fish and pour over the sauce to cover. Sprinkle with the chives, then top with an even layer of cauliflower mash. Use the back of a fork to create a decorative pattern on top, then sprinkle with the remaining cheese. Cook for 30–35 minutes until the top is golden brown.

EASY FISH CAKES WITH SALSA

🍴 serves 4

👨‍🍳 20 mins, plus cooling and chilling   ⏱ 35–40 mins

I used to make fish cakes with salmon, sea bass or cod, but I love these mackerel fish cakes with my salsa. The cooked fish cakes freeze well, so I make a big batch and store some for another day.

Calories: 394 kcal· Carbohydrates: 31 g · Fat: 21 g · Protein: 18 g

3–4 medium potatoes, scrubbed and roughly chopped
10 ounces mackerel fillets
finely grated zest and juice of **1** lime
1 garlic clove, crushed
¾-inch piece of fresh root ginger, peeled and finely grated

small handful of chopped fresh parsley
1 egg, beaten
salt and pepper
2 tablespoons olive oil

Salsa:
2 ripe mangoes, peeled and finely chopped

1 small red onion, finely chopped
1 red pepper, cored, deseeded and finely chopped
handful of fresh parsley, chopped
juice of **1** lime

Serving suggestion:
mixed green salad

1. Cook the potatoes in a saucepan of lightly salted boiling water for 15–20 minutes until tender. Drain well, mash and set aside to cool, covered.

2. Preheat the grill to hot, then cook the mackerel fillets for 5 minutes on each side until cooked through. Set aside to cool.

3. Flake the mackerel into a large bowl. Add the lime zest and juice, garlic, ginger, parsley, egg and cooled mashed potato, season well with salt and pepper and mix thoroughly. Shape the mixture into 8 fish cakes, cover and chill for 20 minutes or overnight.

4. Make the salsa. Place all the ingredients in a bowl, season to taste with salt and pepper and toss to combine.

5. Heat the olive oil in a frying pan over medium heat and cook the fish cakes for about 5 minutes on each side until golden. Serve with the salsa and a mixed green salad.

↪ SWAP

Vegan Swap the mackerel for a can of jackfruit, drained and shredded, and 2 sheets of nori seaweed, broken into strips, to give a mild fishy flavor. Leave out the egg but prepare and cook the "fish cakes" in exactly the same way.

CHICKEN SHISH KEBAB

⛏ serves 4

👨‍🍳 25 mins, plus marinating   ⏱ 15 mins

I'm sure we've all got great memories of a late-night kebab! Now you can re-create that tasty memory at home with your very own chicken shish. It's great for dinner with friends or even a barbecue. The marinade is what makes this dish, yet you'll probably already have all the ingredients in your kitchen cupboard—told you cooking with Krissy is simple!

Calories: 382 kcal · Carbohydrates: 47 g · Fat: 7.8 g · Protein: 27 g

Marinade:
2 tablespoons maple syrup
2 tablespoons olive oil
2 tablespoons soy sauce
1 tablespoon apple cider vinegar
1 teaspoon smoked paprika
1 teaspoon dried oregano
1 teaspoon chili powder

2 chicken breasts, cut into 1 inch cubes
1 large red pepper, cored, deseeded and cut into 1-inch squares
1 large zucchini, cut into chunky slices

1 large onion, cut into 1-inch squares

Garlic sauce:
2 garlic cloves, chopped
½ teaspoon salt
1 cup plain yogurt or coconut yogurt
juice of **1** lemon

Jalapeño sauce:
1 small onion, quartered
¾-inch piece of fresh root ginger, peeled
2 garlic cloves, peeled
1–4 jalapeños (depending on how hot you want it), stalks removed

1 teaspoon coconut sugar or maple syrup
1 tablespoon apple cider vinegar

4 pita breads, warmed
¼ red cabbage, finely shredded
handful of fresh herbs, such as mint or parsley
a few pickled jalapeños
1 lemon, quartered

⊕ Continued on page 148

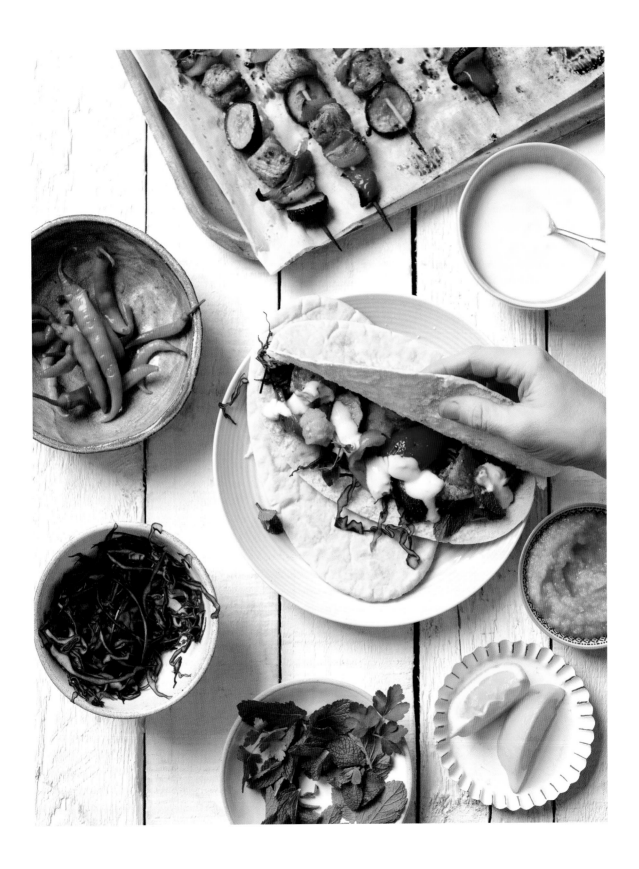

Continued from
page 146

1. Whisk all the marinade ingredients together in a large bowl, add the chicken, red pepper, zucchini and onion, toss to coat and leave in the refrigerator to marinate for 1 hour or overnight.

2. Preheat the oven to 400°F (200°C), and line a baking sheet with parchment paper.

3. Thread the marinated chicken and vegetable pieces onto 4 skewers, alternating the ingredients, and place on the lined baking sheet. Reserve the drained marinade. Cook the kebabs for about 15 minutes until the vegetables are browned and tender and the chicken is cooked through, basting with the reserved marinade halfway through cooking. Alternatively, cook the kebabs in a frying pan over medium heat for about 10 minutes, turning frequently.

4. For the garlic sauce, stir all the ingredients together in a small bowl.

5. For the jalapeño sauce, place all the ingredients in a blender or food processor and blend until smooth.

6. To serve, stuff the pitas with the meat and veggies from the kebabs, shredded cabbage, herbs and pickled jalapeños and drizzle with the garlic sauce and the jalapeño sauce. Squeeze the lemon over the top and enjoy.

⤷ **SWAP**

Vegan Swap the chicken for tempeh pieces or firm tofu and prepare and cook in exactly the same way.

SUNDAY ROAST CHICKEN SHEET PAN

serves 2, generously

15 mins   **1 hour, 20 mins**

Sheet pan dinners are so easy and so mouth-wateringly tasty—exactly what food on a Sunday should be. This is a speedy twist on a traditional Sunday roast with all the flavor and a lot less work.

Calories: 617 kcal · Carbohydrates: 96 g · Fat: 7 g · Protein: 44 g

1 **small** chicken

1 **teaspoon** seasoned salt, plus more to season gravy

black pepper

3 potatoes, peeled and cut into wedges

2 parsnips, peeled and quartered

2 **large** carrots, peeled and quartered

1 **large** red onion, cut into wedges

3 rosemary sprigs

1 lemon, quartered

3 garlic cloves, peeled

olive oil, for drizzling

1 **tablespoon** plain flour

½ cup water

1 chicken stock cube

✍ TIP

Please do not throw away any leftovers. The veggies will be delicious the next day in a Krissy Salad (see page 102), tossed with salad leaves and walnuts and my favorite dressing, while leftover chicken can be used in any number of different ways. Use the chicken carcass to make homemade chicken stock (see page 151).

⊕ Continued on page 151

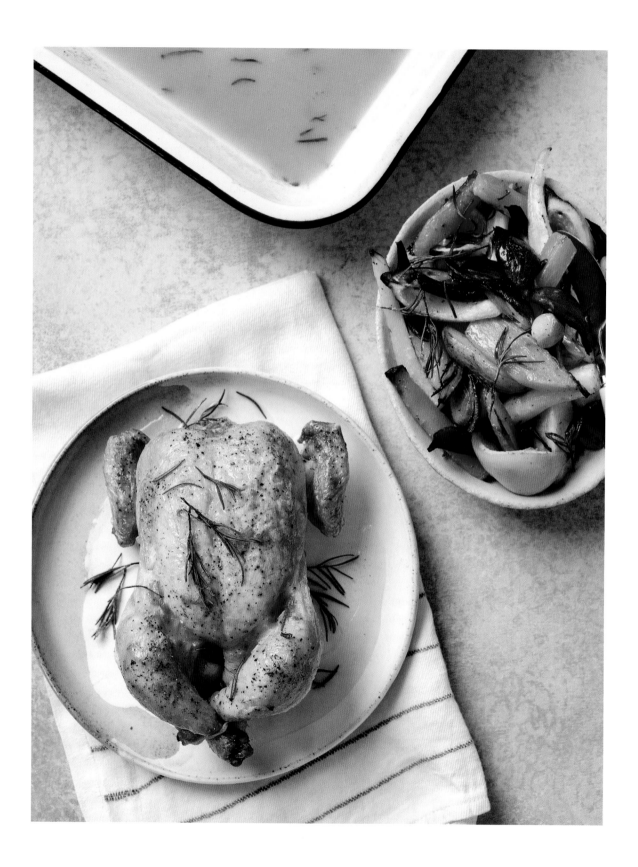

Continued from page 149

1. Preheat the oven to 350˚F (180˚C).

2. Place the chicken in a large roasting pan and sprinkle with the seasoned salt and black pepper. Arrange all the veggies around the chicken, then add the rosemary, lemon and garlic and drizzle with olive oil. Cook for about 1¼ hours, turning the veggies from time to time and basting them and the chicken with the juices, until the veggies are tender and the chicken is cooked through. To make sure the chicken is properly cooked, use a fork to pierce the thickest part of the leg through to the bone—the juices should run clear, not pink. Or use a meat thermometer; it should read 165˚F (74˚C).

3. Once cooked, transfer the chicken to a plate to rest and put the veggies in a bowl ready to serve.

4. Place the roasting pan on a burner over low heat and stir in the flour to make a paste, then whisk in the measured water and crumble in the stock cube, whisking continually as the gravy thickens. If you like your gravy thin, add a little more water. Simmer the gravy for 2 minutes, then season to taste and pour into a gravy boat.

5. Carve the chicken and serve with the roasted veggies and gravy.

☑ TIP

If you like a little spice, add 4 cardamom pods, a few cloves, 1 teaspoon of chili powder and a sprinkle of cinnamon to the roasting pan before cooking and toss the chicken and veggies in the spices to coat. It will really change the flavors up, giving a more Mediterranean vibe.

↪ SWAP

Vegan *Cook the roasted veggies in exactly the same way and serve with Stuffed Peppers (see page 101) or your favorite vegan sausages.*

CHICKEN STOCK

🍴 **makes 2 liters**
⏱ **2 hours**

A roasted chicken carcass makes great stock, which can be used to add flavor to soups, gravies, stews and sauces, so don't throw away the bones.

1 roasted chicken carcass, including bones, skin and leftover meat
1 celery stick
1 carrot, scrubbed
1 onion, halved (skin on)
2 bay leaves
8 cups water

1. Place all the ingredients in a large saucepan over high heat and bring to a boil. Reduce the heat and simmer for 2 hours, then allow to cool. Once cooled, drain the liquid and freeze in portions of about 2 cups for up to 3 months.

CHICKEN KORMA

🍴 serves 2, generously

👨‍🍳 15 mins   ⏱ 25 mins

I love going out for Indian food, but I love making it at home even more. People sometimes think it's too complicated, but you can make a delicious, flavorful curry with ingredients you probably already have in your kitchen cupboard. Once you've sorted your curry base, you can make it your own with chicken, fish or tofu—or get creative with your veggies and meat and share your recipes with me too! Serve the korma on a bed of rice, sprinkled with sliced almonds.

Calories: 483 kcal · Carbohydrates: 21 g · Fat: 19.4 g · Protein: 35 g

2 chicken breasts, cubed
2 tablespoons olive oil
1 onion, chopped
2 garlic cloves, chopped
¾-inch piece of fresh root ginger, peeled and chopped

1 teaspoon chili powder
1 teaspoon garam masala
1 teaspoon turmeric
1 teaspoon ground coriander
½ cup water
½ cup tomato purée
1 cup ground almonds

¼ cup + 1 tablespoon low-fat plain yogurt
salt and pepper

Serving suggestion:
cooked rice
sliced almonds

1. Season the chicken well. Heat 1 tablespoon of olive oil in a frying pan over medium-high heat, add the chicken and cook, stirring, for 10 minutes, or until golden.

2. Meanwhile, heat the remaining olive oil in a large saucepan over medium-low heat, add the onion, garlic and ginger and cook for about 5 minutes until softened. Add in the spices and cook for another 2 minutes, stirring. Add in the measured water and tomato purée and bring to a boil. Reduce the heat, cover and simmer for 5 minutes.

3. Add the chicken to the sauce and simmer for 10 minutes, or until the chicken is cooked through. Stir in the ground almonds and yogurt and season to taste. Serve in bowls on a bed of rice, sprinkled with sliced almonds.

⤷**SWAP**

Fish Swap the chicken for 2 cooked white fish fillets, such as bass or cod.
Vegan Swap the chicken for 1 cup of cooked firm tofu.

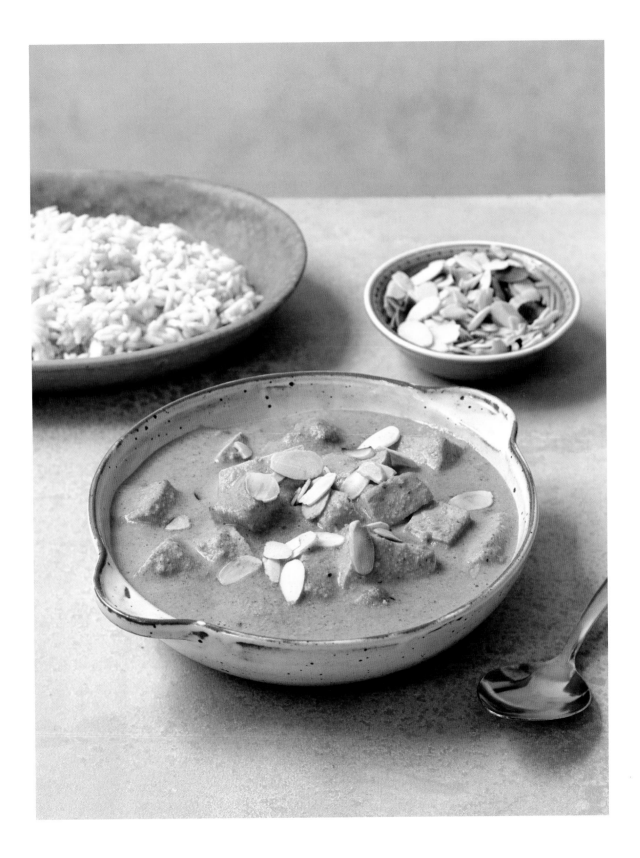

PIZZA

makes 4 pizzas

20 mins **30–35 mins**

I love ordering pizza in—it's my favorite takeout—but I love making pizza even more! People think pizza can take hours, but this super-easy recipe will have your pizza ready quicker than a takeout. Follow the basic recipe below to make the pizza bases and tomato sauce, then choose your toppings to complete your pizza.

Calories: 312 kcal · Carbohydrates: 59 g · Fat: 3 g · Protein: 10 g

Dough:
2½ cups self-rising flour, plus extra for dusting
1¼ cups plain yogurt or coconut yogurt

Tomato sauce:
3 tablespoons olive oil
1 large onion, chopped
2 garlic cloves, crushed
2 x 14.5-ounce cans diced tomatoes

1 tablespoon tomato purée
1 teaspoon dried oregano
1 teaspoon sugar
salt and pepper

1. Preheat the oven to 400°F (200°C), and line 2 baking sheets with parchment paper.

2. Place the dough ingredients in a mixing bowl and mix with a spoon until combined, then knead briefly with your hands until it forms a smooth dough. Divide into 4 equal pieces and roll out on a lightly floured surface to make 4 pizza bases, about 6 inches across.

3. Transfer to the lined baking sheets and cook for 10 minutes, then set aside.

4. Meanwhile, make the tomato sauce. Heat the olive oil in a large saucepan over medium-low heat, add the onion and garlic and cook for about 5 minutes until softened. Add the remaining sauce ingredients and bring to a boil, then lower the heat and simmer for 15 minutes. Season with salt and pepper to taste.

5. Spread a few tablespoons of tomato sauce over each of the part-baked pizza bases, then add your desired toppings. Return to the oven and cook for 10–15 minutes until the cheese is gooey and golden.

TIP

Freeze any leftover dough or tomato sauce for next time by placing in an airtight container or freezer bag in the freezer—they can be stored for up to 4 weeks.

MARGHERITA TOPPING

serves 4 **5 mins**

♡ **Pizza plus topping**

Calories: 388 kcal · Carbohydrates: 59.4 g · Fat: 8.8 g · Protein: 15.7 g

1 ball of mozzarella cheese, drained and chopped   **handful** of pitted black olives (optional)

HAWAIIAN BBQ TOPPING

serves 4 **5 mins**

♡ **Pizza plus topping**

Calories: 455 kcal · Carbohydrates: 63.3 g · Fat: 9.8 g · Protein: 19.5 g

1 ball of mozzarella cheese, drained and chopped   **8-ounce can** chopped pineapple in juice, drained
4 slices of ham, chopped   barbecue sauce, to serve

PEPPERONI TOPPING

serves 4 **5 mins**

♡ **Pizza plus topping**

Calories: 525 kcal · Carbohydrates: 59.3 g · Fat: 17.8 g · Protein: 23.2 g

1 ball of mozzarella cheese, drained and chopped   **4 ounces** pepperoni slices

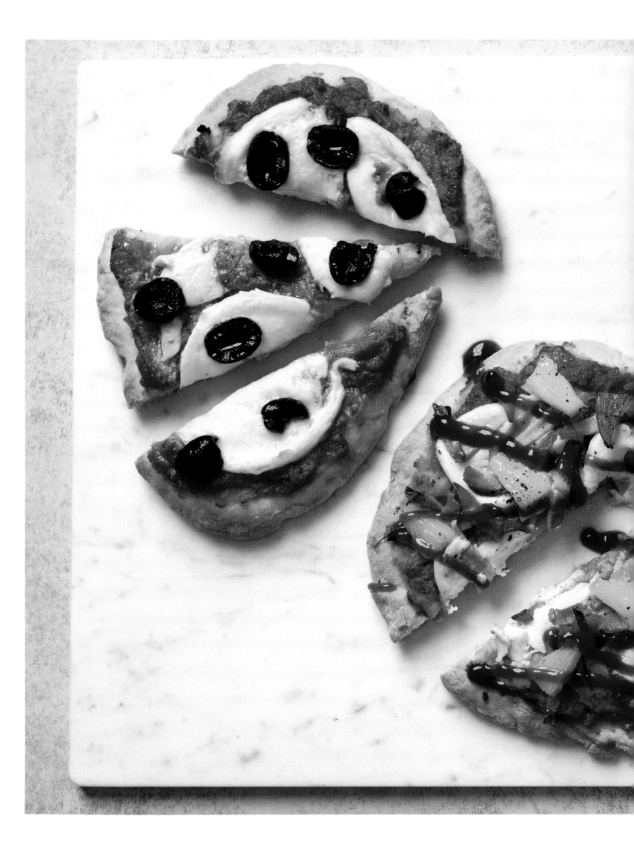

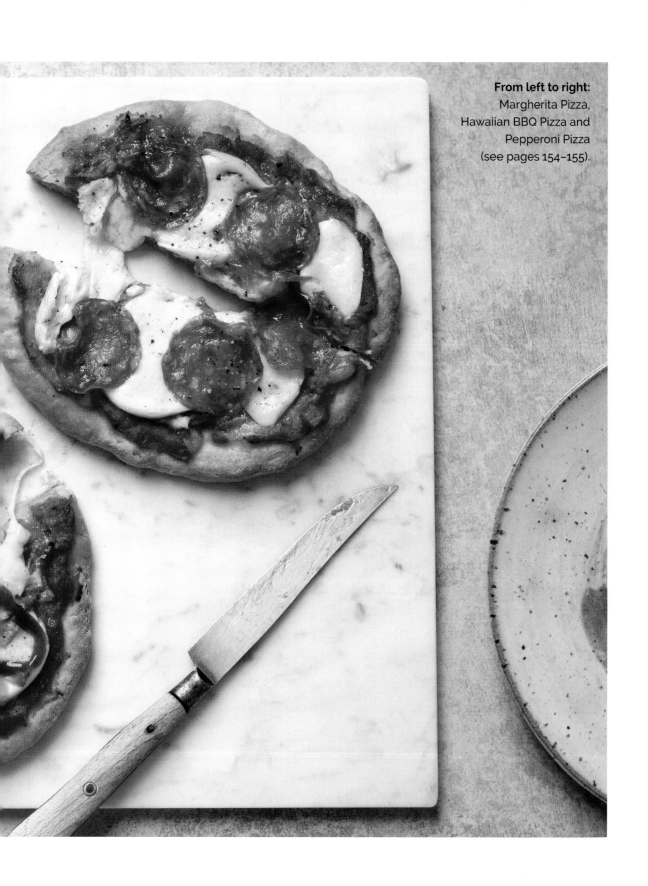

From left to right:
Margherita Pizza,
Hawaiian BBQ Pizza and
Pepperoni Pizza
(see pages 154–155).

NO-PASTA LASAGNE

¶¶ serves 4

👨‍🍳 20 mins   ⏱ 1 hour, 15 mins

Now pizza is a firm favorite, but nothing—and I mean nothing—beats lasagne! I love layers of food, and lasagne can be as many layers as you want. I got creative, used all the veggies in my fridge and voilà: here is your no-pasta lasagne. Of course you can use pasta sheets if you'd prefer, but try it without first. Trust me, you will love all the flavor.

Calories: 767 kcal · Carbohydrates: 40 g · Fat: 44 g · Protein: 54 g

olive oil, for greasing
2 zucchini, thinly sliced
   lengthways
1 eggplant, thinly sliced
   lengthways
salt

Bolognese sauce:
1 teaspoon olive oil
1 onion, finely chopped
2 garlic cloves, finely chopped
14 ounces lean ground beef
1½ cups mushrooms, roughly
   chopped
14.5-ounce can diced tomatoes
1 bay leaf
1 tablespoon tomato purée
splash of Worcestershire sauce
small glass of red wine (optional)
salt and white pepper

Béchamel sauce:
1 tablespoon butter or
   coconut oil
2 tablespoons all-purpose
   flour
1¾ cups milk of your choice
½ cup Cheddar cheese, grated

¾ cup Cheddar cheese, grated
1 crust of bread, grated
crisp green salad, to serve

1. Preheat the oven to 400°F (200°C), and lightly grease 2 baking sheets.

2. Arrange the zucchini and eggplant slices in a single layer on the baking sheets. Season with salt and cook for about 10 minutes until softened. Set aside.

3. Meanwhile, make the Bolognese sauce. Heat the oil in a large saucepan over low heat and fry the onion and garlic for a few minutes until softened. Turn up the heat a little and add the ground beef. Cook for about 5 minutes, stirring, then add the mushrooms and cook for 1 minute more.

4. Add the tomatoes, bay leaf, tomato purée, Worcestershire sauce and red wine, if using. Season well with salt and white pepper, bring to a boil, reduce the heat and simmer for 15 minutes.

⊕ Continued on page 160

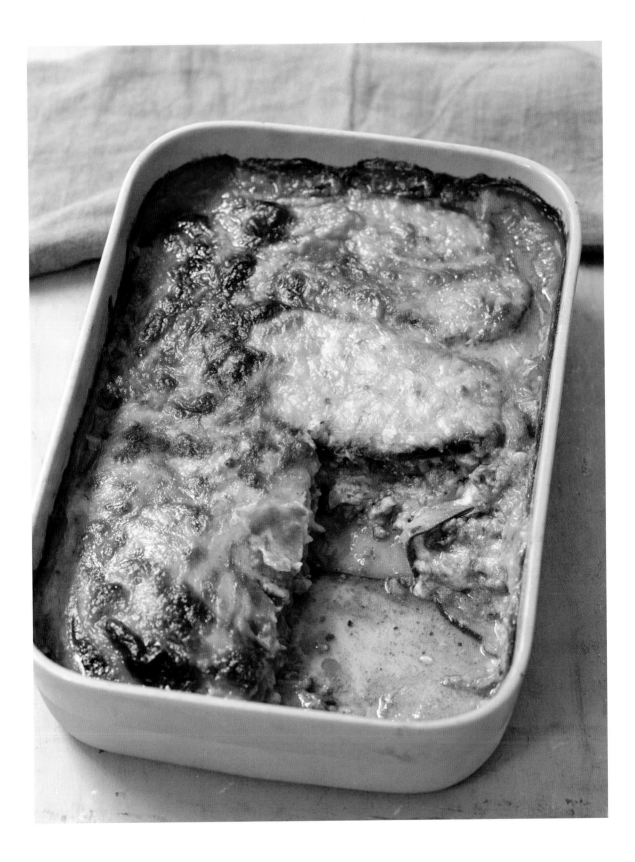

Continued from
page 158

5. For the béchamel, melt the butter or coconut oil in a saucepan over a low heat. Add the flour and incorporate with a whisk. Allow the mixture to bubble for 2 minutes, then gradually add the milk, whisking continuously to remove any lumps. Simmer gently for 3 minutes, stirring frequently, then add the cheese and season well with salt and white pepper.

6. Use a paper towel to pat both sides of the zucchini and eggplant slices to remove any moisture. Spoon half the Bolognese sauce into a large ovenproof dish and top with half the veggies in an even layer. Next spoon over half the béchamel. Repeat the layers with the remaining ingredients, then top with the cheese and bread crumbs. Cook for about 45 minutes until bubbling and golden. Serve immediately with a crisp green salad.

7. Any leftovers can be stored in individual portions in an airtight container in the freezer for up to 4 weeks.

⌐→ **SWAP**

Vegan Swap the ground beef for vegan mince and swap the grated cheese in the béchamel for 2 tablespoons of nutritional yeast. Top the lasagne with bread crumbs and 2 tablespoons of nutritional yeast, omitting the cheese.

THE KRISSY BURGER

¶¶ serves 4

🍳 10 mins   ⏱ 15 mins

This is the ultimate burger, the ONLY burger you'll be feasting on from now on! This is my recipe for burger patties and burger sauce. Choose from the list of serving options below to stack your burger the way you like it. If you want a feast, then you can serve these with Loaded Sweet Potato Fries (see page 105), Raw Slaw (see page 162) or one of my milkshakes (see page 180).

Calories: 413 kcal • Carbohydrates: 10 g • Fat: 25 g • Protein: 35.5 g

---

½ onion, finely chopped
1 teaspoon garlic granules
½ teaspoon smoked paprika
1 egg
1¼ pounds lean ground beef
1 tablespoon
   Worcestershire sauce
1 tablespoon soy sauce
salt and pepper

Burger sauce:
1 tablespoon low-fat
   mayonnaise
1 tablespoon ketchup
1 teaspoon yellow or grain
   mustard
1 tablespoon vinegar from
   a jar of pickles
½ onion, finely chopped

Serving suggestions:
toasted brioche burger buns
sliced pickles
sliced tomato
sliced cheese
shredded lettuce
barbecue sauce
fried bacon
sliced red onion

☑ TIP
The recipe makes 4 burger patties—you may want a double burger if you are really hungry, or you can freeze any uncooked patties for another day.

⊕ Continued on page 162

Continued
from page 161

1. Place all the burger ingredients in a mixing bowl, season well with salt and pepper and combine thoroughly with your hands until well mixed. Divide the mixture into 4 portions and shape into burgers, about ¾-inch thick. Transfer to a plate, cover and place in the refrigerator until needed—this will help to firm them up.

2. Preheat the grill to hot, then cook the burgers for about 15 minutes, turning halfway, until browned and just cooked through. If using cheese, lay the slices over the burgers for the final 1 minute of cooking time to melt them.

3. Meanwhile, whisk all the burger sauce ingredients together in a small bowl. Taste and add a little more of any of the ingredients if you like.

4. Now, stack your burger using any of the serving suggestions. I do mine in this order: bun, burger sauce, burger, pickles, lettuce, tomato, sliced red onion, bun top and ENJOY.

5. Freeze any uncooked burger patties and use within 1 month.

↪ SWAP

Vegan Swap the meat for a 15-ounce can of kidney beans, rinsed and drained. Mash the beans with 1 teaspoon of smoked paprika, then follow the burger recipe above.

RAW SLAW

🍴 serves 4   👨‍🍳 15 mins

Calories: 57 kcal · Carbohydrates: 12 g · Fat: 1.1 g · Protein: 1.1 g

1 large carrot, scrubbed and grated
1 apple, cored and grated
½ red onion, finely sliced
⅛ red cabbage, finely sliced
1 tablespoon low-fat mayonnaise
1 tablespoon low-fat yogurt
small handful of fresh parsley, finely
  chopped
salt and pepper

1. Place all the ingredients in a large bowl, season well with salt and pepper and toss to coat in the mayonnaise and yogurt.

2. Any leftovers can be stored in an airtight container in the refrigerator for up to 3 days.

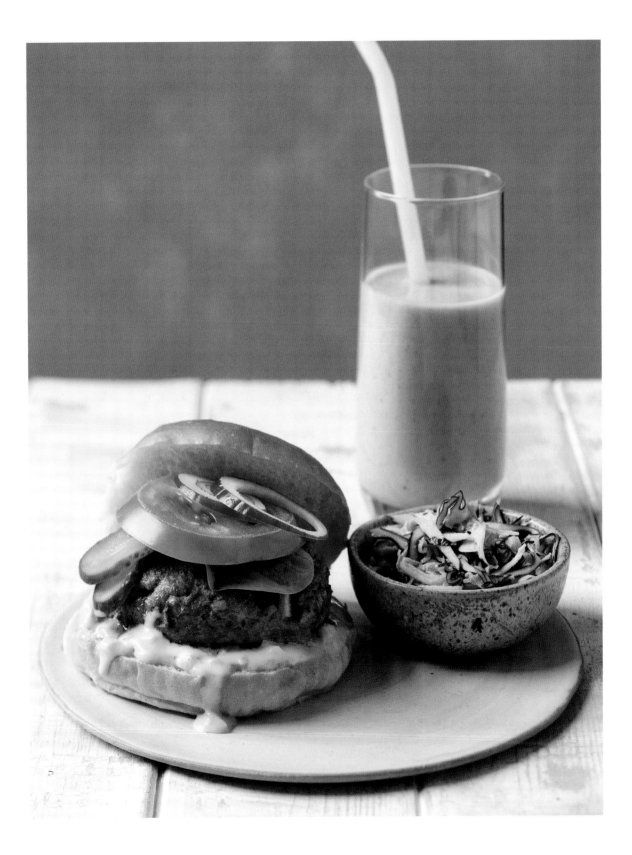

DESSERT

BERRY CRUMBLE

🍴 serves 6

👨‍🍳 15 mins   ⏱ 35 mins

This crumble tastes so warm and sweet—it really hits the spot! I make this for my friends and family when I have them all over for dinner. It works so well with Vanilla Nice Cream (see page 168).

Calories: 413 kcal · Carbohydrates: 52.9 g · Fat: 22.2 g · Protein: 6.3 g

2 large apples, peeled, cored and chopped
2 cups fresh or frozen berries
¼ cup brown sugar
1 teaspoon ground cinnamon
1 tablespoon lemon juice
2 cloves
2 tablespoons water

Crumble topping:
1½ cups pecans or walnuts
6 pitted dates
1¾ cups rolled oats
1 teaspoon ground cinnamon
3 tablespoons brown sugar or coconut sugar
1 tablespoon coconut oil

Serving suggestion:
Vanilla Nice Cream (see page 168) or yogurt

1. Preheat the oven to 350˚F (180˚C).

2. Place the apples, berries, sugar, cinnamon, lemon juice, cloves and measured water in a saucepan over high heat. Bring to a boil, stirring, then reduce the heat to low and cook for 10 minutes, or until the apples are soft. Remove from the heat and set aside.

3. Meanwhile, place all the topping ingredients in a food processor and pulse until well combined.

Alternatively, if you don't have a food processor, chop the nuts and dates roughly and place in a mixing bowl. Add the remaining topping ingredients and use your hands to mix them to a crumbly consistency.

4. Spoon the fruit filling into an ovenproof dish and top with the crumble mixture. Bake for about 20 minutes until the top is golden and the fruit is bubbling away underneath. Serve with Vanilla Nice Cream or yogurt.

STICKY TOFFEE PUDDING

¶¶ serves 8

♔ 10 mins   **⏱ 25–30 mins**

This dessert makes me feel like I'm at a restaurant finishing off a delicious meal, but I can have it whenever I like with this mouth-watering recipe. The toffee sauce isn't a standard recipe, but I know you'll love it as much as I do. Any leftovers can be eaten cold as a cake or will freeze well for another day.

Calories: 277 kcal · Carbohydrates: 39 g · Fat: 11 g · Protein: 4.2 g

⅔ cup pitted dates
⅓ cup boiling water
1 teaspoon vanilla extract
3 tablespoons coconut oil, softened, plus extra for greasing

⅓ cup maple syrup
2 large eggs, beaten
¾ cup self-rising flour
½ teaspoon baking soda

Toffee sauce:
⅔ cup pitted dates
1 cup coconut milk
pinch of salt
1 teaspoon vanilla extract

1. Preheat the oven to 350°F (180°C), and line an 8-inch square brownie pan with parchment paper.

2. Put the dates in a heatproof bowl and pour over the boiling water. Leave for 5 minutes to soften, then mash with the liquid until smooth, using a fork. Stir in the vanilla and set aside.

3. Place the coconut oil, maple syrup, eggs, flour and baking soda in a mixing bowl and beat thoroughly with an electric mixer on high speed until smooth. Stir in the mashed dates.

4. Pour the mixture into the prepared pan and cook for 25–30 minutes until risen and firm to the touch.

5. Meanwhile, place all the sauce ingredients in a blender or food processor and blend until smooth, adding more coconut milk if the mixture is too thick. Serve the sauce poured over the hot pudding.

6. Freeze any leftover pudding in an airtight container for up to 6 weeks.

☑ TIP
This pudding also tastes great with a scoop of Vanilla Nice Cream (see page 168).

⤷ SWAP
Vegan Swap the eggs for 2 teaspoons of chia seeds soaked in ½ cup of water for 10 minutes before use.

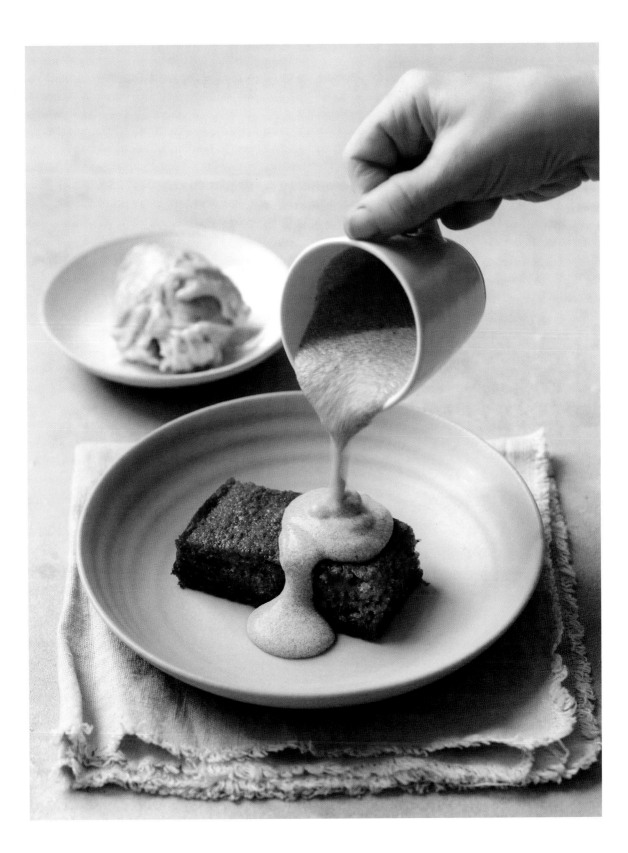

NICE CREAMS

Yes, you can actually make your own ice cream at home with all the flavor you crave! It takes just 10 minutes to blitz up and an hour to freeze. You could even put the mixture in lollipop molds for friends and family. These lighter ice creams can be served on their own or alongside a pudding, such as Sticky Toffee Pudding (see page 166). Keep a stash of peeled ripe bananas in an airtight container in the freezer to make a batch whenever you want some.

VANILLA NICE CREAM

🍴 serves 4   👨‍🍳 10 mins

Calories: 47 kcal · Carbohydrates: 10 g · Fat: 0 g · Protein: 0.7 g

2 large ripe bananas, frozen
¼ cup almond milk,
   or other milk of your choice
2 teaspoons vanilla extract

1. Place all the ingredients in a blender or food processor and blend on high speed for 1–2 minutes until smooth, stopping to scrape down the sides every so often.

2. Serve immediately or transfer to an airtight container and freeze for 1–2 hours until firm enough to scoop like ice cream.

✒ TIP

If you freeze your Nice Cream for longer than 1–2 hours, it will become too hard and will need to be thawed. Just defrost for 20 minutes to soften before serving.

PEANUT BUTTER NICE CREAM

🍴 serves 4   👨‍🍳 10 mins

Calories: 239 kcal · Carbohydrates: 25 g · Fat: 13 g · Protein: 5.2 g

2 large ripe bananas, frozen
2 tablespoons peanut butter

⅔ cup almond milk, or other milk
of your choice
½ cup chocolate chips

1. Place all the ingredients, except the chocolate chips, in a blender or food processor and blend on high speed for 1–2 minutes until smooth, stopping to scrape down the sides every so often. If it's too thick, add a little more milk. Stir in the chocolate chips.

2. Serve immediately or transfer to an airtight container and freeze for 1–2 hours until firm enough to scoop like ice cream.

CHOCOLATE NICE CREAM

🍴 serves 4   👨‍🍳 10 mins

Calories: 137 kcal · Carbohydrates: 13 g · Fat: 5.7 g · Protein: 6.5 g

2 large ripe bananas, frozen
¾ cup cocoa powder
1 teaspoon vanilla extract

½ cup almond milk, or other milk
of your choice
chocolate chips, to serve

1. Place all the ingredients in a blender or food processor and blend on high speed for 1–2 minutes until smooth, stopping to scrape down the sides every so often. If it's too thick, add a little more milk.

2. Serve immediately, sprinkled with chocolate chips, or transfer to an airtight container and freeze for 1–2 hours until firm enough to scoop like ice cream.

ETON MESS

🍴 serves 2, with spare meringues
👨‍🍳 10 mins, plus cooling   ⏱ 40 mins

My favorite summer dessert, perfect on a hot day or after a barbecue.
You can buy ready-made meringues, but these are so easy to make and
taste so much better.

Calories: 201 kcal · Carbohydrates: 29 g · Fat: 4.3 g · Protein: 15 g

Meringues:
4 egg whites at room temperature
¼ cup confectioners' sugar
1 teaspoon vanilla extract
¼ teaspoon cream of tartar
2 teaspoons apple cider vinegar
small pinch of salt

1¼ cups strawberries, hulled and
halved
1 cup plain yogurt
toasted almond slices, to serve

1. Preheat the oven to 275°F (140°C), and line 2 baking sheets with parchment paper.

2. Place the egg whites in a mixing bowl and beat with an electric mixer on high speed until stiff peaks form. Slowly add the remaining meringue ingredients and fold together until combined.

3. Spoon the mixture onto the baking sheets, making 4 mounds of about 3 inches in diameter. Bake for 20 minutes, then reduce the oven temperature to 225°F (110°C), and bake for another 20 minutes.

4. Turn the oven off but leave the meringues in the oven to cool for at least 2 hours, or overnight if possible.

5. Carefully remove the meringues from the parchment paper and break a meringue per person into pieces. Layer the broken meringue in serving bowls with the strawberries and yogurt. Top with toasted almond slices and serve immediately.

6. Store the leftover meringues in an airtight container for up to 4 weeks.

☑ TIP
Leftover meringues are delicious with fresh mango and coconut yogurt for a quick pudding.

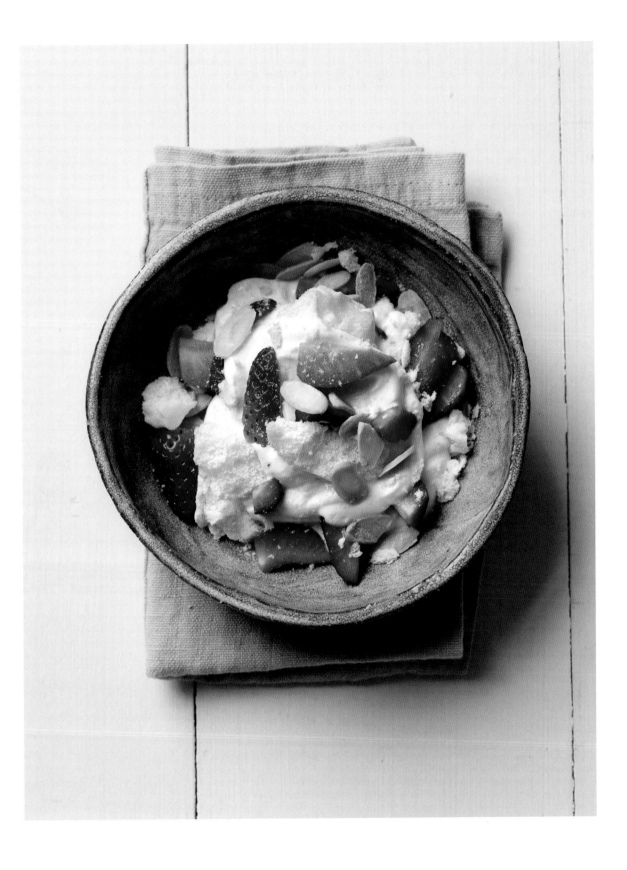

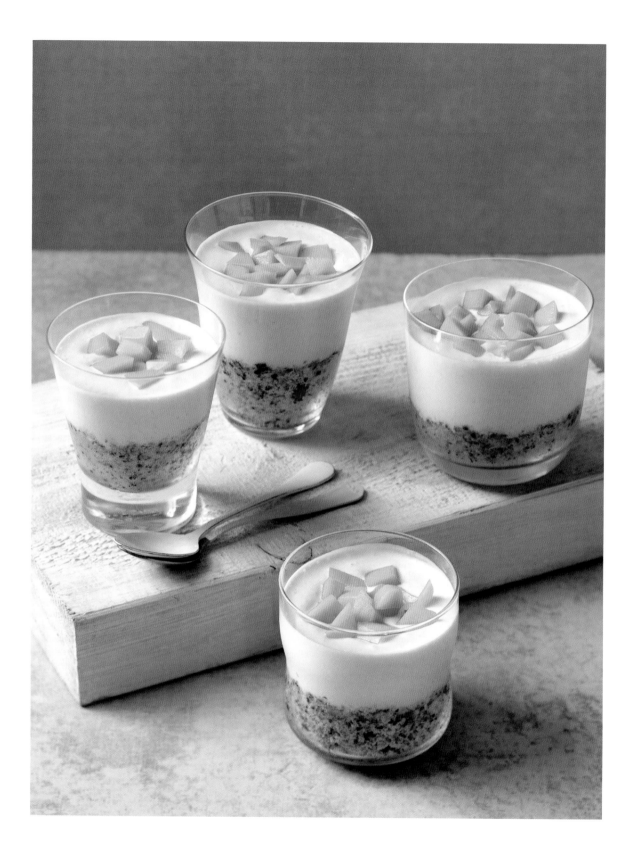

MANGO CHEESECAKE POTS

serves 6

15 mins, plus chilling

Mango has to be one of my favorite fruits; it always makes me feel like I'm on vacation. You just can't go wrong with it. Here it tops my cheesecake pots—you just won't want your pot to end. These taste so good and need to chill for only an hour—if you can wait that long!

Calories: 346 kcal · Carbohydrates: 20 g · Fat: 24 g · Protein: 10 g

Base:
1 cup almonds
10 pitted dates
⅔ cup shredded coconut
1 tablespoon coconut oil, melted
½ teaspoon vanilla extract

Filling:
¾ cup reduced-fat coconut milk

¾ cup reduced-fat cream cheese,
  at room temperature
2 tablespoons maple syrup
¼ cup half-fat crème fraîche
squeeze of lemon juice
1 teaspoon vanilla extract

1 fresh mango, peeled and diced,
  or **¾ cup** mango chunks

1. Place all the ingredients for the base in a blender or food processor and pulse until well mixed and finely chopped. Divide between 4 small jars or glasses and press down to form an even layer. Chill in the refrigerator while you make the filling.

2. Place all the ingredients for the filling in a blender or food processor and blend until smooth and airy.

Divide between the jars or glasses, using a spatula to scrape the sides of the blender so you don't waste any.

3. Top with the chopped mango and chill in the refrigerator for 1 hour before serving.

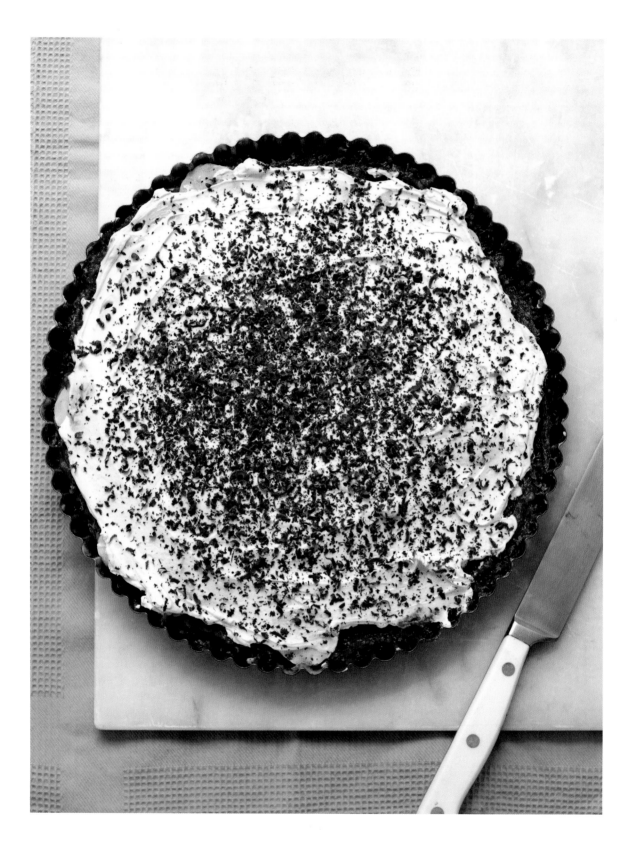

BANOFFEE PIE

🍴 serves 12

👨‍🍳 30 mins, plus chilling

I love pie, especially after dinner. This tastes unreal! Your friends and family will love it, and it's very easy to make. Any leftovers can be frozen in portions for up to 6 weeks—a great dessert to have in the freezer for when you fancy something sweet.

Calories: 373 kcal · Carbohydrates: 36 g · Fat: 22 g · Protein: 4.8 g

Crust:
1⅓ cups shredded coconut
1 cup pecans
1 cup pitted dates
1 tablespoon maple syrup
pinch of salt

Raw caramel:
2⅓ cups pitted dates, soaked in hot water for 5 minutes
3 tablespoons peanut or almond butter
pinch of sea salt
1 teaspoon vanilla extract

2 large bananas, sliced
¾ cup whipping cream, whipped
2 squares of dark chocolate, grated

1. Place all the crust ingredients in a blender or food processor and blend until well combined. Tip the mixture into a 9-inch pie pan, then press evenly over the base and up the sides with your fingers to form a crust. Firm up by placing in the refrigerator for 1 hour or the freezer for 15 minutes.

2. For the caramel, drain the dates and place in a blender or food processor with the remaining caramel ingredients and blend until smooth, stopping to scrape down the sides of the bowl if necessary.

3. Spread the caramel evenly over the chilled crust. Chill for about 1 hour to set.

4. Arrange the sliced bananas on top of the chilled caramel and top with whipped cream. Decorate with the grated chocolate.

⤷SWAP
Vegan Swap the whipped cream for a 14-ounce can of coconut milk. Chill in the refrigerator overnight, then whip it until thick.

CHOCOLATE POTS

🍴 makes 4 large pots
👨‍🍳 10 mins, plus setting

Of course I'm going to have a chocolate dessert—but this is my own twist.
These chocolate pots are so quick and easy to make and so nutritious too.
I love curling up with my dog, Buttons, my favorite film and one (or two)
of these desserts every once in a while.

Calories: 282 kcal · Carbohydrates: 24.7 g · Fat: 22.2 g · Protein: 3.2 g

2 ripe avocados
2 tablespoons coconut oil, melted
3 tablespoons raw honey
½ teaspoon vanilla extract
4 tablespoons cocoa powder
2 pinches of salt
1 teaspoon ground cinnamon (optional)

1. Place all the ingredients in a blender or food processor and blend until silky and smooth.

2. Pour into 4 glasses and leave to set for 1 hour before serving.

BROWNIES

makes 12 brownies

10 mins, plus cooling   **25 mins**

Brownies aren't just for dessert, these are great for snacking too. I love one with my coffee—but then I love anything sweet with my coffee! These are quick to make and easy to store.

Calories: 233 kcal · Carbohydrates: 19.9 g · Fat: 15.4 g · Protein: 4.5 g

1½ cups dark chocolate (at least 70% cocoa solids), broken into pieces

3 eggs

2 tablespoons coconut oil, melted

½ cup brown sugar

1 teaspoon vanilla extract

1 tablespoon cocoa powder

⅔ cup plain wholemeal flour

1 teaspoon baking powder

pinch of salt

1. Preheat the oven to 400°F (200°C), and line an 8-inch square brownie pan with parchment paper.

2. Place the chocolate in a heatproof bowl over a small saucepan of gently simmering water, making sure the water does not touch the bowl. Stir occasionally until melted, then set aside.

3. Place the eggs, coconut oil, sugar and vanilla extract in a mixing bowl and beat with an electric mixer on high speed for about 5 minutes until thick. Add the cocoa, flour, baking powder and salt and gently fold in, using a large metal spoon. Add the melted chocolate and gently fold in until well mixed.

4. Spoon into the lined brownie pan and bake for 20 minutes, then set aside to cool in the pan. Remove from the pan and cut into 12 squares. The insides will be lovely and moist.

5. Store any leftover brownies in an airtight container for up to 7 days.

☑ TIP
These brownies taste great served with a scoop of Vanilla Nice Cream (see page 168).

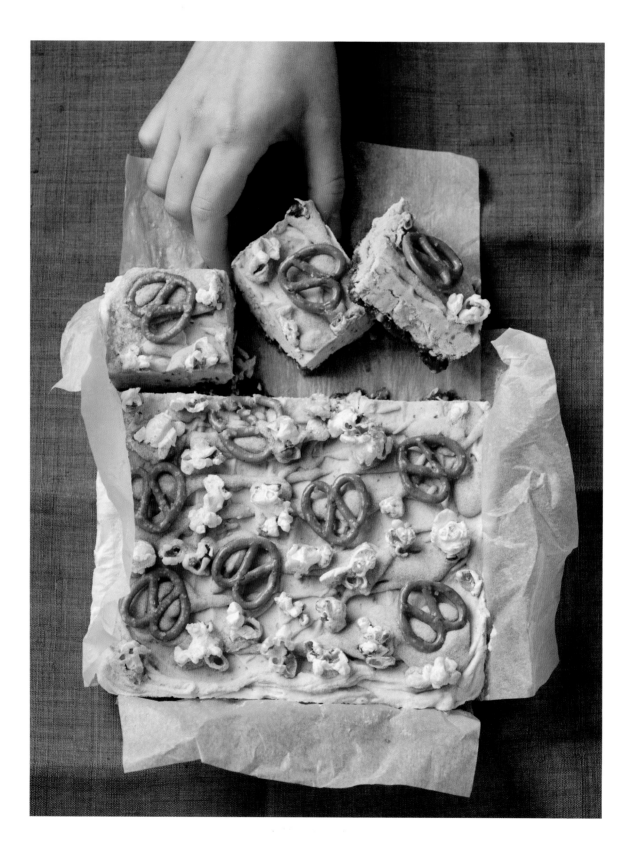

SALTED CARAMEL SQUARES

🍴 **makes 12 squares**
👨‍🍳 **10 mins, plus freezing**

Who doesn't love salted caramel? After chocolate, it has to be my favorite flavor. These squares are great for dessert or a sweet snack— just try not to eat them all at once!

Calories: 261 kcal · Carbohydrates: 20 g · Fat: 16 g · Protein: 7 g

---

Base:
1⅓ cups pitted dates, soaked in hot water for 5 minutes
¾ cup almonds
¼ teaspoon sea salt

2 cups reduced-fat cream cheese
1 teaspoon vanilla extract
1 tablespoon maple syrup
⅔ cup pitted dates, soaked in hot water for 5 minutes
2 teaspoons sea salt flakes
⅔ cup double cream

Serving suggestions:
½ quantity of Toffee Sauce (see page 166)
salted pretzels
popcorn

---

1. Line an 8-inch square brownie pan with parchment paper.

2. For the base, drain the dates and place in a blender or food processor with the remaining base ingredients and blend to form a soft crumble. Transfer the mixture to the lined brownie pan and press down to form an even base layer.

3. Place the cream cheese, vanilla extract and maple syrup in a bowl and beat with an electric mixer until smooth.

4. Drain the dates and place in a blender or food processor with the sea salt flakes and cream and blend until smooth. Scrape the date mixture into the cream cheese mixture and whisk again until light and fluffy. Spoon the mixture over the base layer in the pan and spread out evenly.

5. Drizzle the toffee sauce over the cheese mixture and top with the pretzels and popcorn. Place the pan in the freezer for 1 hour to set, then turn out and cut into 12 portions.

6. Freeze any leftovers for up to 4 weeks.

MILKSHAKES

My shakes are full of goodness and sweetness—they are nutritious, filling and make great on-the-go snacks. They are also the perfect dessert on a hot summer's day. Chocolate peanut butter is my absolute favorite, but I've included a sweet strawberry one as I know it's loved by so many—enjoy!

CHOCOLATE PEANUT BUTTER SHAKE

🍽 makes 1 milkshake   👨‍🍳 5 mins

Calories: 494 kcal · Carbohydrates: 45 g · Fat: 25 g · Protein: 18 g

1 large ripe banana
2 tablespoons peanut butter
3 pitted dates
1 tablespoon cocoa powder

1¼ cups almond milk, or other milk of your choice
6 ice cubes
pinch of salt

1. Place all the ingredients in a blender or food processor and blend until smooth.

STRAWBERRY SHAKE

🍽 makes 1 milkshake   👨‍🍳 5 mins

Calories: 328 kcal · Carbohydrates: 57 g · Fat: 5 g · Protein: 8.1 g

1 large ripe banana
1½ cups frozen strawberries
1¼ cups almond milk, or other milk of your choice

1 tablespoon maple syrup
1 tablespoon natural yogurt
1 teaspoon vanilla extract
6 ice cubes

1. Place all the ingredients in a blender or food processor and blend until smooth.

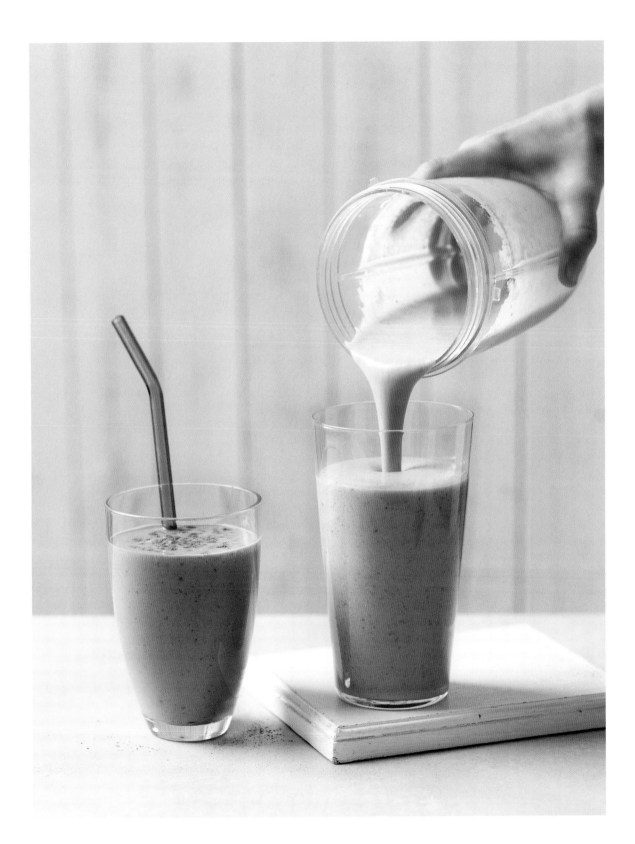

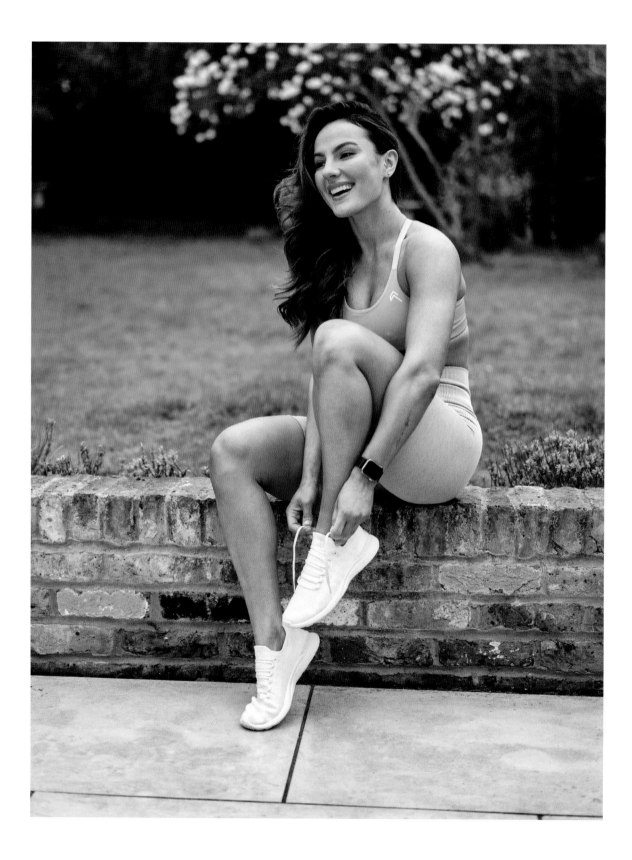

3

MOVE
MOVE
MOVE

YOUR EXERCISE GUIDE

When I first started going to the gym, I knew absolutely nothing about working out. Apart from running on a treadmill and doing a few squats and lunges, I did nothing else. In fact, I didn't actually step foot in the gym for two months after joining—I had a lot going on, but more than anything, I didn't know what I was doing there. I wish I had had a guide like this, and I am proud to share my knowledge and best workouts with you to kick-start your fitness regime.

Back when I started, home workouts and gym workouts were two very different things. If you worked out outside the gym, you pretty much just went running or maybe went to a class here and there—everything outside the gym was very cardio based. Research, experience and lifestyle changes have taught us a lot—that you can get an effective resistance- and strength-based workout at home too. The workouts in this section have been designed to be done anywhere at any time. You can be confident that you will be getting stronger and stronger day by day. Each workout is designed to get you in the mindset to really believe you are doing this for your happiness and your health—nothing and no one else matters. All you need is this guide, a mat and a dumbbell, if you have one.

Using the Exercises in This Book

I love training with weights and my body weight. To help you build up your strength, I've put a range of exercises together, which you can mix and match to create the best workout for you.

You will find the exercises in this book divided into ten groups. Groups One to Five focus on the upper body and abs, while Groups Six to Ten focus on the lower body. All the exercises complement one another.

You can:

- Simply choose six exercises for your workout and follow the number of repetitions provided on each page. For a full workout, repeat the exercises for three sets (or four if you want a real challenge), with a 60-second rest between each set.

- Stick to an upper-body workout with the exercises in Groups One to Five.

- Stick to a lower-body workout with the exercises in Groups Six to Ten.

- Combine all the different types of exercises for a full-body workout.

- Alternatively, create a HIIT, Ladder or AMRAP workout based on the instructions provided on pages 186–190.

- If you fancy a real challenge, make sure to add an exercise or two from the Full-Body Finisher (see pages 244–249) to the end of your workout.

Don't forget to warm up by skipping for 5 minutes, running on the spot for 5 minutes or completing the mobility exercises on pages 192–194—you just need to get the blood flowing through your body. The most important thing is to do what works best for you and your routine. When putting your weekly plan together, just select your exercises so you know what you're doing before you begin. And you're good to go!

A note on repetitions and sets: repetitions, or "reps," refer to the number of times you repeat a particular exercise or movement. The number of rounds of repetitions you complete for a particular exercise is known as a "set." Repetitions and sets are important because they help you time and plan your workouts effectively and efficiently.

Safety note: To avoid the risk of slipping and injury, when completing exercises that involve using a chair, make sure that the chair is placed against the wall.

HOW DO I PUT A WORKOUT TOGETHER?

There are so many different ways to work out, and it can feel overwhelming—I totally understand, as this is how I felt when I first started going to the gym. I'd look around and see people doing all different types of workouts: in the weights section I'd see some people working through ladder sets and some hitting a personal best. In the cardio section, I'd see people smashing a high-intensity interval training (HIIT) workout and some people working through steady-state cardio sessions. The most important thing to remember is to find a style of workout that suits you—try everything and mix it up too.

To help you out, here is an overview of some of the different types of workouts you might want to try when putting your exercises together. Just remember: always warm up before and cool down after your workout.

HIIT

HIIT stands for high-intensity interval training—performing high-intensity exercises (usually cardio based) for short intervals, with rests in between. The most standard intervals are 30 seconds of work with a 30-second rest in between, for 10–15 minutes.

You could try a range of exercises, from jumping squats and burpees combined with low-resistance tricep extensions or lunges. HIIT training is great for building stamina and body-weight strength, and it's perfect if you're short on time.

HIIT

Upper body

Choose 1 exercise from each group		
EXERCISE	TIME	REST
Group 1	30 secs	30 secs
Group 2	30 secs	30 secs
Group 3	30 secs	30 secs
Group 4	30 secs	30 secs
Group 5	30 secs	30 secs
Repeat 3 times		

Lower body

Choose 1 exercise from each group		
EXERCISE	TIME	REST
Group 6	30 secs	30 secs
Group 7	30 secs	30 secs
Group 8	30 secs	30 secs
Group 9	30 secs	30 secs
Group 10	30 secs	30 secs
Repeat 3 times		

Full body

Choose 1 exercise from each group		
EXERCISE	TIME	REST
Groups 1–5	30 secs	30 secs
Groups 6–10	30 secs	30 secs
Groups 1–5	30 secs	30 secs
Groups 6–10	30 secs	30 secs
Full-body finisher	30 secs	30 secs
Repeat 3 times		

15-minute abs

Choose 1 exercise from each group		
EXERCISE	TIME	REST
Group 3	30 secs	30 secs
Group 5	30 secs	30 secs
Group 1	30 secs	30 secs
Group 3	30 secs	30 secs
Group 5	30 secs	30 secs
Repeat 3 times		

AMRAP

AMRAP stands for "as many reps as possible." This type of workout is a great and efficient way of building strength as it pushes your body to the maximum in a set amount of time.

To perform an AMRAP workout, choose three exercises. Do 12–15 reps of each one with no rest in between and repeat as many times as possible for 5 minutes. Choose three different exercises and do the same again, before repeating the whole workout from the beginning. You can play around with your exercises and put them together according to the muscle groups you want to focus on.

What Are Pre-Workout Supplements?

Pre-workout supplements contain a mix of different ingredients such as caffeine, creatine, amino acids, B vitamins and more, which are designed to boost your energy and performance levels. It's important to check the ingredients of your pre-workout formula and, if you're unsure, check with a nutritionist or doctor to see if it will work for you.

If you like working out in the morning, your breakfast or pre-workout snack should be supplement enough. It needs to be a good mix of fats, proteins and carbohydrates (think eggs, avocado, oatmeal, peanut butter). If you tend to work out after work or school, this is where pre-workout supplements can help boost your energy levels. I tend to take my pre-workout supplement 30–60 minutes before my workout and sometimes keep sipping during my workout too.

The most important thing is to stay hydrated and keep your body fueled so you feel energized throughout your workout.

AMRAP SETS

Upper body

Choose 3 exercises from Groups 1–5	12–15 reps of each
Repeat as many times as possible in 5 mins	
Choose another 3 exercises from Groups 1–5	12–15 reps of each
Repeat as many times as possible in 5 mins	
Repeat once from the beginning	

Lower body

Choose 3 exercises from Groups 6–10	12–15 reps of each
Repeat as many times as possible in 5 mins	
Choose another 3 exercises from Groups 6–10	12–15 reps of each
Repeat as many times as possible in 5 mins	
Repeat once from the beginning	

Full body

Choose 3 exercises from Groups 1–5	12–15 reps of each
Repeat as many times as possible in 5 mins	
Choose 3 exercises from Groups 6–10	12–15 reps of each
Repeat as many times as possible in 5 mins	
Repeat once from the beginning	

LADDERS

Ladders

The way to perform ladders is to choose one exercise—for example, squats—and begin by doing 10 reps with a 10-second rest, then dropping to 9 reps with a 10-second rest, then 8 reps and so on until you reach 1 rep. Alternatively, start with 1 rep and work up to 10 reps.

Ladders are intense, so I would recommend doing them only once a week with each muscle group. This type of format can take some time and therefore is best performed if you have more time for your workout.

Choose your exercise	
10 reps	10-sec rest
9 reps	10-sec rest
8 reps	10-sec rest
7 reps	10-sec rest
6 reps	10-sec rest
5 reps	10-sec rest
4 reps	10-sec rest
3 reps	10-sec rest
2 reps	10-sec rest
1 rep	10-sec rest

WARM-UP & MOBILITY

Warming up your body and mind is super important before you start working out. You can do this either by going for a quick run (outside or on a treadmill), skipping (my absolute favorite) or by doing a mobility warm-up.

Mobility is a little different to stretching. Mobility warm-ups are dynamic, active (you're moving while you're doing them), and they warm up your muscles and joints. They get the blood flowing round your body, helping your body to feel supple before you begin lifting. Cardio warm-ups are absolutely fine, but I find mobility warm-ups work really well when you're going to lift weights. Why?

- They activate the muscles for maximum output and efficiency during your workout.

- They help increase your range of motion when exercising (for example, you might squat lower or deepen your lunge during your workout).

- They prevent injury.

My favorite mobility exercises can be found on pages 192–194.

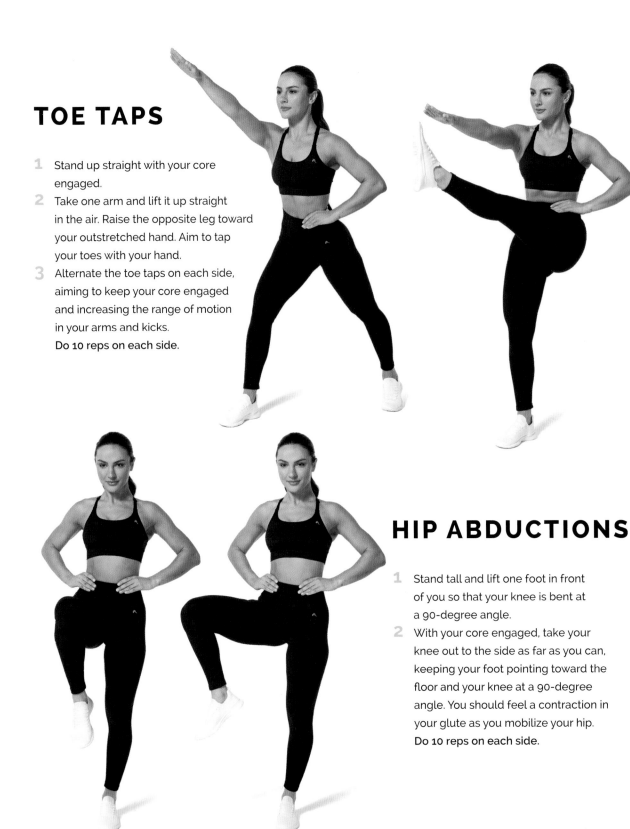

TOE TAPS

1. Stand up straight with your core engaged.
2. Take one arm and lift it up straight in the air. Raise the opposite leg toward your outstretched hand. Aim to tap your toes with your hand.
3. Alternate the toe taps on each side, aiming to keep your core engaged and increasing the range of motion in your arms and kicks.
   Do 10 reps on each side.

HIP ABDUCTIONS

1. Stand tall and lift one foot in front of you so that your knee is bent at a 90-degree angle.
2. With your core engaged, take your knee out to the side as far as you can, keeping your foot pointing toward the floor and your knee at a 90-degree angle. You should feel a contraction in your glute as you mobilize your hip.
   Do 10 reps on each side.

SQUAT ROTATIONS

1. Sit in a deep squat—point your feet outward to stabilize your body. Cross your arms to touch your shoulders.
2. Slowly bring your right knee down to hover above the floor while twisting on the balls of your feet. Return to the deep squat.

Do 5 reps on each side.

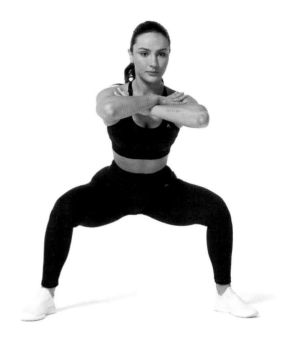

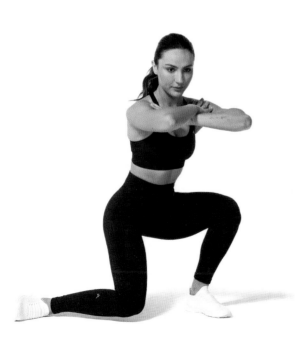

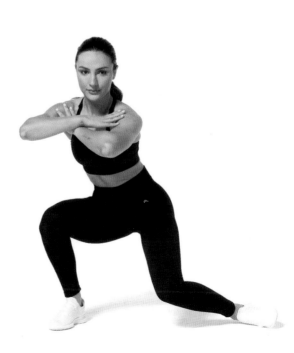

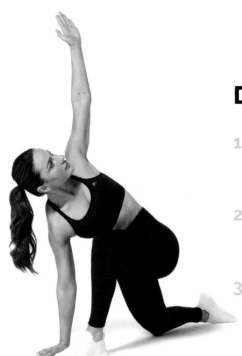

DEEP LUNGE ROTATION

1 Stand with feet hip distance apart, then take a big step back with your right leg, bending both knees and lunging down until your back knee touches the floor. You should feel a stretch in your quads and hip flexor.

2 Place your right hand next to your left foot and lift your left arm up to the side, following it around with your eyes, as if you are trying to reach for the sky. Your arms will almost form a straight line.

3 Take a nice, big deep breath in as you return to the starting position.
Do 5 reps on each side.

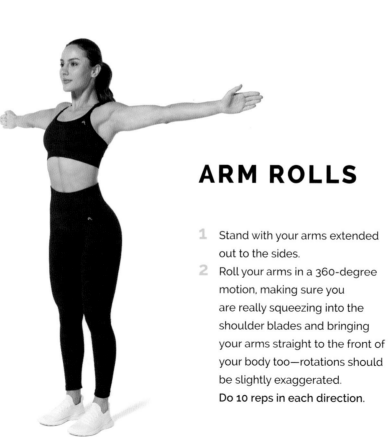

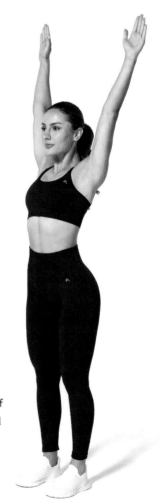

ARM ROLLS

1 Stand with your arms extended out to the sides.

2 Roll your arms in a 360-degree motion, making sure you are really squeezing into the shoulder blades and bringing your arms straight to the front of your body too—rotations should be slightly exaggerated.
Do 10 reps in each direction.

COOLING DOWN AFTER A WORKOUT

After a workout, our heart rate is high and muscles are warm. Usually, we tend to sit down to rest or shower and get back to our day-to-day activities. However, cooling down post-workout is important as it returns your heart rate to resting, which prevents feelings of dizziness, light-headedness and headaches. Plus, stretching can help alleviate muscle soreness and prevent injuries.

I tend to cool down with some stretches to give me a few minutes to take deep breaths. Giving yourself 5–10 minutes to just breathe, stretch and relax can do wonders for your mind and body—I can never finish a workout without it! Here are some of my favorite cooldown exercises.

HAMSTRING STRETCHES

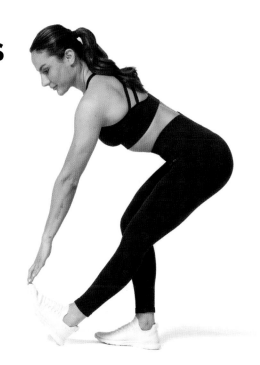

1   Stand up straight, place one foot out in front of the other, then lean backward by hinging at your hips.
2   Come up onto your front-foot heel and reach your hand to your toes to extend the stretch into your hamstring. Keep your front leg straight and back leg slightly bent.
3   Hold for 20 seconds and repeat on the other side.

QUAD STRETCHES

1. Stand tall with your feet hip width apart. Pull your abdominals in and relax your shoulders. You can hold onto a wall for stability if you like.
2. Bend your left leg, bringing your heel toward your bum, and grasp your left foot with your left hand. Push your hips forward slightly to really feel a stretch down the front of your leg.
3. Hold for 20 seconds and repeat on the other side.

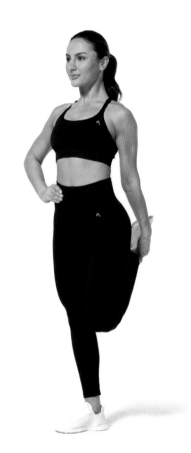

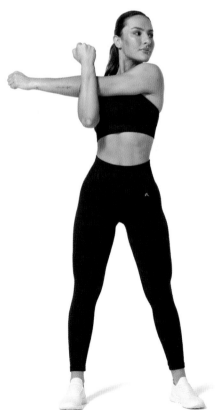

SHOULDER STRETCHES

1. Bring your left arm across your chest and lift your right arm to support it.
2. Using your right arm, pull your left elbow toward your right shoulder to feel a stretch across your upper back and shoulders. Turn your head to look in the opposite direction to your arm.
3. Hold for 20 seconds, then repeat on the other side.

LOWER-BACK TWIST

1 Sit up on a mat with your legs straight out in front of you.
2 Take your left foot over your right leg and place it just by your knee. Place your left hand on the floor behind you to help with balance.
3 Twist your body to face your left leg and use your right hand to pull in your bent left knee. You should feel a stretch run through your lower back.
4 Hold for 10–15 seconds, then repeat on the other side.

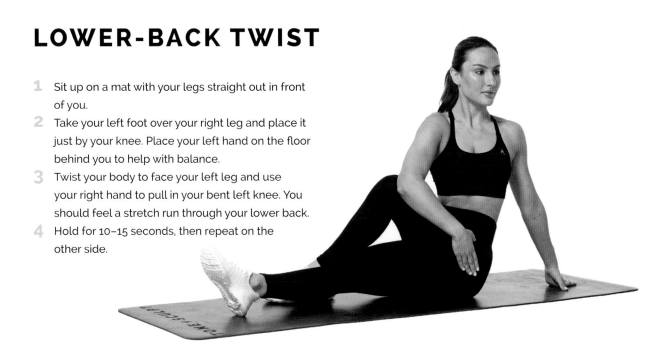

PIGEON STRETCHES

1 Begin on your hands and knees. Place your left ankle near your right wrist so your shin is lying behind your hands. Extend your right leg back so that your knee and right foot are resting on the floor.
   Press through your fingertips as you lift your torso away from your thigh.
2 Lengthen the front of your body and release your tailbone back toward your heels. Work on squaring your hips by balancing your weight between them. The aim is to keep them as close to the floor as possible. To relax a little more into it, you can let your body fall forward—facedown, arms stretched out in front of you—to feel a nice stretch run through your back too.
3 Hold for 30 seconds, then repeat on the other side.

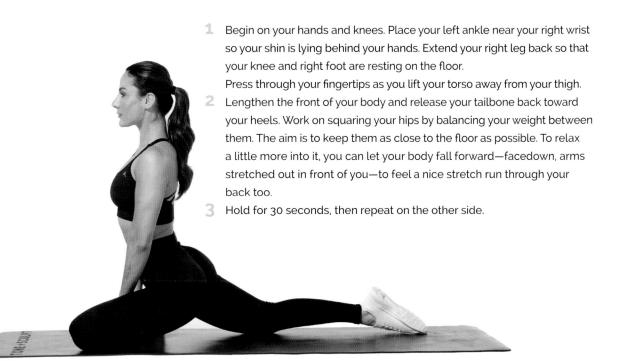

KEY MUSCLES & FORM

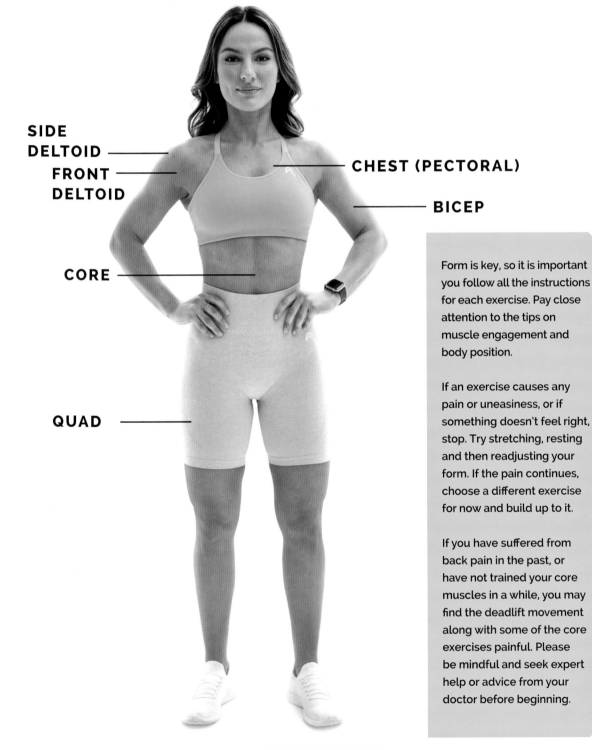

SIDE DELTOID

FRONT DELTOID

CHEST (PECTORAL)

BICEP

CORE

QUAD

Form is key, so it is important you follow all the instructions for each exercise. Pay close attention to the tips on muscle engagement and body position.

If an exercise causes any pain or uneasiness, or if something doesn't feel right, stop. Try stretching, resting and then readjusting your form. If the pain continues, choose a different exercise for now and build up to it.

If you have suffered from back pain in the past, or have not trained your core muscles in a while, you may find the deadlift movement along with some of the core exercises painful. Please be mindful and seek expert help or advice from your doctor before beginning.

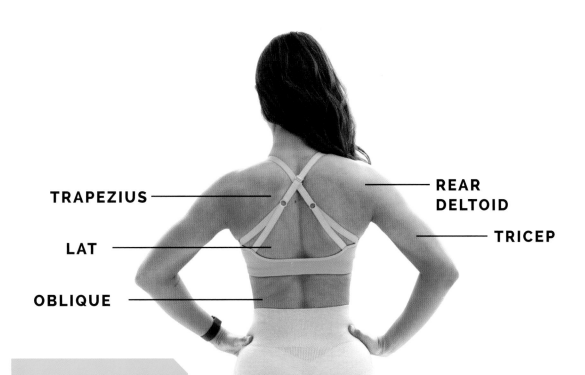

TRAPEZIUS

LAT

OBLIQUE

REAR DELTOID

TRICEP

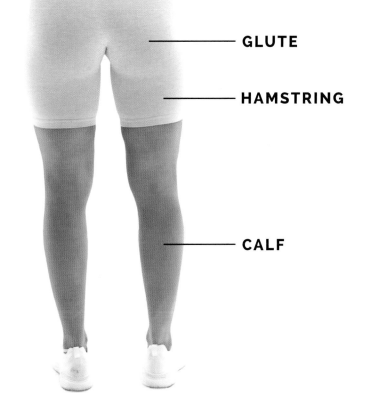

GLUTE

HAMSTRING

CALF

Here I've identified major muscles and muscle groups that will come up in your workouts.

When performing the exercises in this book, you will mainly target the primary muscles mentioned but will also recruit and engage the secondary muscles.

It's good to know which muscles we're hitting to target mind-muscle connection: research tells us that if we really think about the muscles we're targeting in a workout, we're more likely to exercise them!

PLANK

PRIMARY MUSCLES USED: **core**
SECONDARY MUSCLES USED: **triceps, trapezius, lats, glutes, hamstrings, calves**

The plank is a perfect strength-building and conditioning exercise—it benefits the whole body. To prevent hunching the shoulders and losing tension in your core, push your heels back—you'll be able to hold the position for longer. If you find it hurts your back at all, simply go down onto your knees. For a high plank, lift up onto your hands with arms straight and hands slightly wider than shoulder distance apart.

1   Lie on a mat on your front with your body raised on your forearms, making sure your elbows are directly underneath your shoulders.

2   Place your feet close together behind you, pushing your heels back.

3   Make sure your back is in line with your neck and shoulders. There should be no arching in the back—you should be in a straight line.

4   Keep your core engaged and hold this position for 30 seconds.

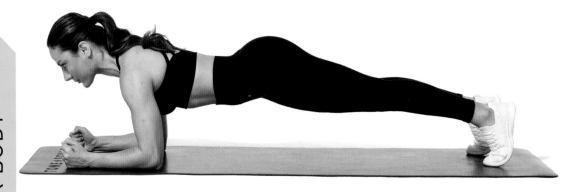

SHOULDER TAPS

PRIMARY MUSCLES USED: **core**
SECONDARY MUSCLES USED: **deltoids**

This is a great variation on the plank. The fact that you can't sway from side to side adds that extra challenge for your core and mind!

1   Start in a high plank position on your hands with arms straight and hands slightly wider than shoulder distance apart.

2   Keeping your feet hip distance apart, rest back on the balls of your feet.

3   Keep your core engaged. Make sure your back is in line with your neck and shoulders. There should be no arching in the back—you should be in a straight line.

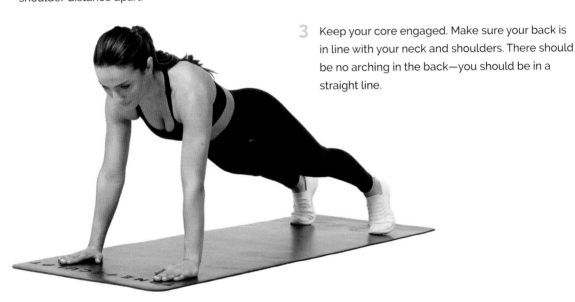

4   Take one hand and touch the opposite shoulder. Try not to move your hips—keep everything still by keeping your core engaged.

5   Repeat with the other hand.
    Do 6–8 reps on each side.

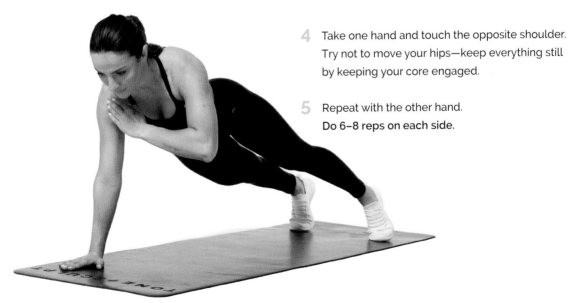

PLANK ROTATION

PRIMARY MUSCLES USED: **core, obliques**
SECONDARY MUSCLES USED: **triceps**

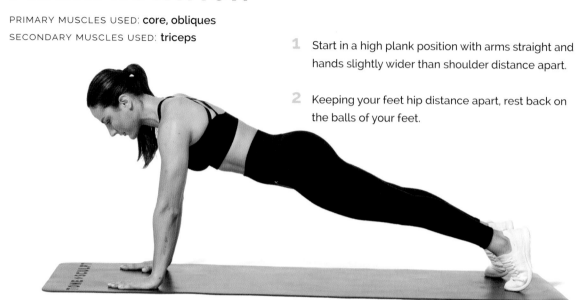

1 Start in a high plank position with arms straight and hands slightly wider than shoulder distance apart.

2 Keeping your feet hip distance apart, rest back on the balls of your feet.

3 Keep your core engaged. Make sure your back is in line with your neck and shoulders. There should be no arching in the back—you should be in a straight line.

4 Take one hand off the floor and lift it up to the side, following it around with your eyes, as if you are trying to reach for the sky. Your arms will almost form a straight line.

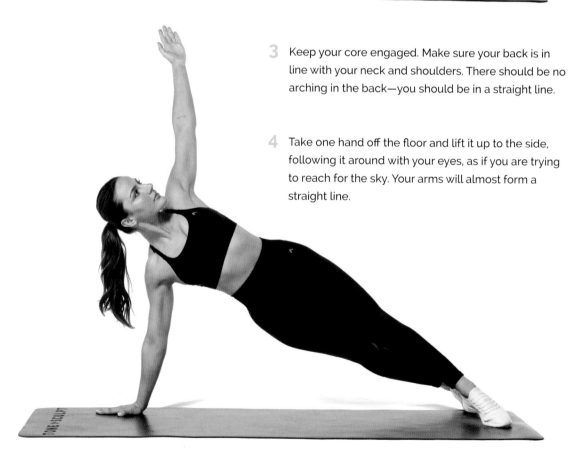

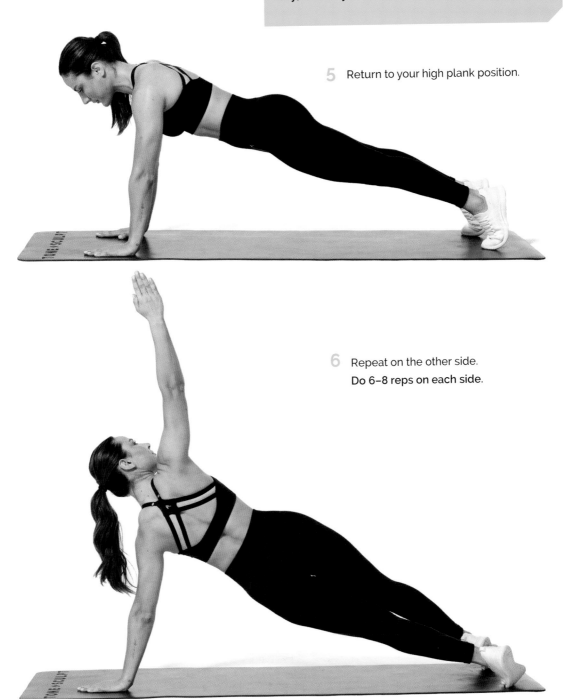

Plank rotations add an extra challenge to your balance and core—you'll definitely feel it the next day, and maybe even after that!

5   Return to your high plank position.

6   Repeat on the other side.
     Do 6–8 reps on each side.

COMMANDO

PRIMARY MUSCLES USED: **core**
SECONDARY MUSCLES USED: **chest, triceps**

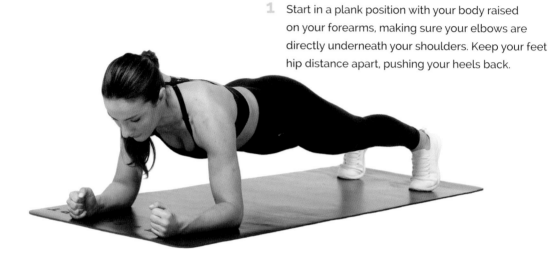

1 Start in a plank position with your body raised on your forearms, making sure your elbows are directly underneath your shoulders. Keep your feet hip distance apart, pushing your heels back.

2 Keep your core engaged. Make sure your back is in line with your neck and shoulders. There should be no arching in the back.

3 Push up on your left hand so your left arm is straight.

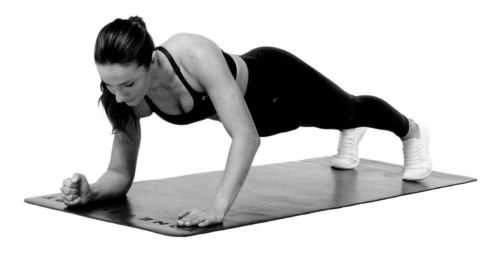

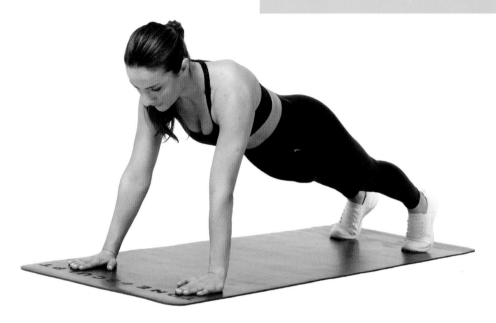

4   Push up on your right hand, lifting up into a high plank position. Try not to sway with your hips.

5   Pause and then go back down onto your left forearm, followed by the right.

6   Repeat, starting with the opposite arm. **Do 6–8 reps on each side.**

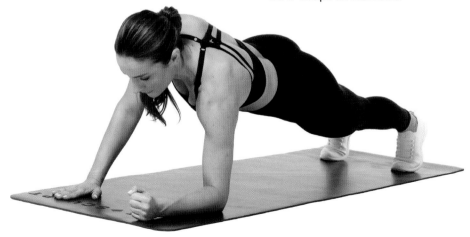

PUSH-UP TWO WAYS

PRIMARY MUSCLES USED: **chest**
SECONDARY MUSCLES USED: **core, triceps**

1 Start in a kneeling plank position with hands slightly wider than shoulder distance apart. Keep your knees together and feet either resting on the floor or raised up behind you, whichever feels more comfortable.

2 Keep your core engaged and your back, neck and shoulders in a straight line.

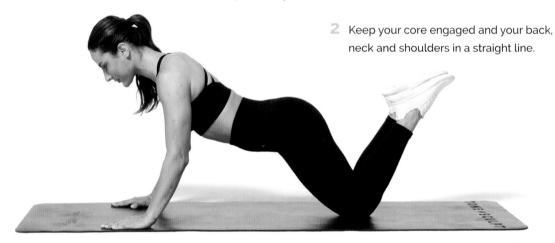

3 Bending your elbows, slowly lower your body down to the floor, until you are hovering just above it. Try to keep your elbows tucked in throughout.

4 As you exhale, push back up into the starting position.
Do 12–15 reps.

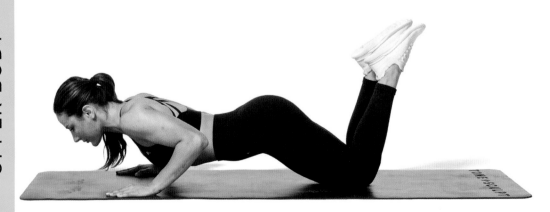

Push-ups are one of the best body-weight strength-building exercises. They are such a challenge and an achievement—which you will learn to love! Once you have mastered this exercise on your knees, try the full-body movement below. If you struggle with the full-body movement or it causes any pain, continue to perform the exercise on your knees instead.

1   Start on the floor in a high plank position, with arms straight and your hands slightly wider than shoulder distance apart. Keep your feet hip distance apart, placed behind you, and maintain a position on the balls of your feet.

2   Keep your core engaged and your back, neck and shoulders in a straight line.

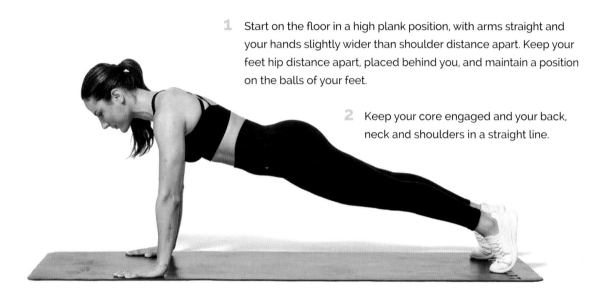

3   Bending your elbows, slowly lower your body down to the floor, until you are hovering just above it. Try to keep your elbows tucked in throughout.

4   As you exhale, push back up into the starting position.
    Do 12–15 reps.

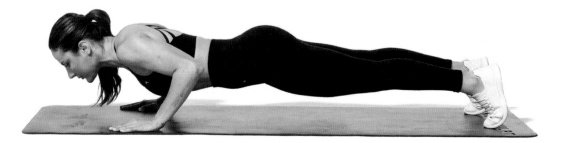

MOUNTAIN CLIMBER

PRIMARY MUSCLES USED: **core, chest**
SECONDARY MUSCLES USED: **quads**

You can pretty much add this move to all workouts. To challenge your stamina and cardiovascular strength, perform the move more quickly, but slow it down to really fire up your core.

1   Start on the floor in a high plank position, with arms straight and your hands slightly wider than shoulder distance apart. Keep your feet hip distance apart, placed behind you, and maintain a position on the balls of your feet.

2   Bring one knee into your chest, then return to the starting position.

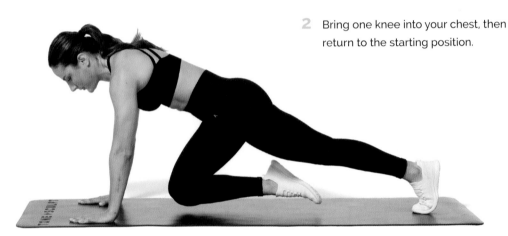

3   Repeat with the other knee, feeling your core crunch as you alternate your legs. **Do 6–8 reps on each side.**

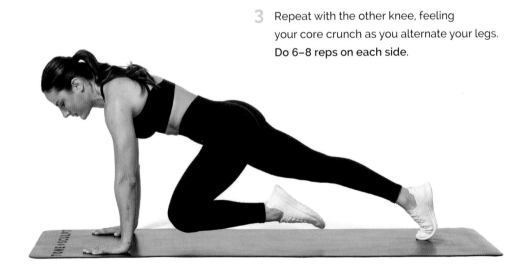

KNEELING DIAMOND PUSH-UP

PRIMARY MUSCLES USED: **chest**
SECONDARY MUSCLES USED: **triceps, trapezius**

This exercise is great for strengthening your triceps and chest. It's a real game changer for your upper body, and I absolutely love it—it makes me feel so strong!

1   Start on your knees with hands close together, your two index fingers and thumbs forming a diamond shape directly under your chin.

2   Keep your knees together and feet either resting on the floor or raised up behind you, whichever feels more comfortable.

3   Keep your core engaged and your back, neck and shoulders in a straight line.

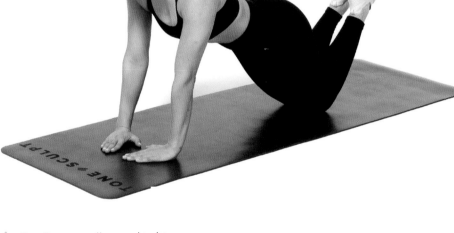

4   Bending your elbows, slowly lower your body down to the floor, until you are hovering just above it. Try to keep your elbows tucked in throughout.

5   As you exhale, push back up into the starting position. **Do 12–15 reps.**

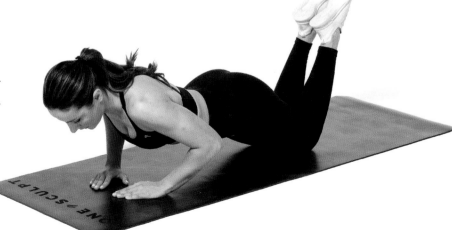

WIDE-TO-NARROW PUSH-UP

PRIMARY MUSCLES USED: **triceps, chest**
SECONDARY MUSCLES USED: **core, biceps**

1 Start in a high plank position with arms straight but with your hands positioned at the edge of the mat. Keep your feet hip distance apart, placed behind you, and maintain a position on the balls of your feet. Keep your core engaged and your back, neck and shoulders in a straight line.

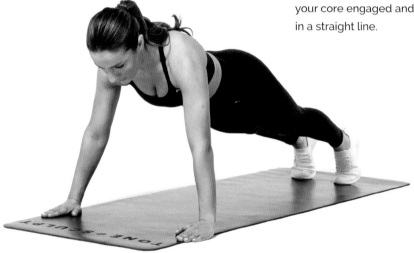

2 Bending your elbows, slowly lower your body down to the floor until you are hovering just above it. Try to keep your elbows tucked in throughout. As you exhale, push back up into the starting position.

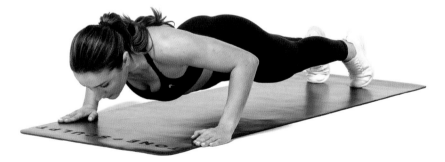

Wide-to-narrow push-ups challenge all areas of your upper body—chest, core, biceps and triceps. This will really leave your upper body feeling it for days. A great way to build upper-body strength and stamina.

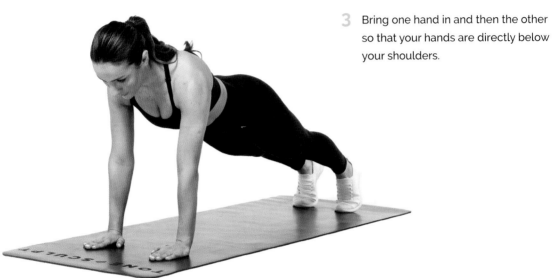

3   Bring one hand in and then the other so that your hands are directly below your shoulders.

4   Push down into a narrow push-up, and then return to the start position.

5   Widen your hands and repeat the movement, alternating wide and narrow push-ups.
    Do 12–15 reps.

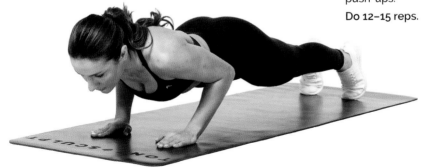

PLANK HIP DIP

PRIMARY MUSCLES USED: **core, obliques**
SECONDARY MUSCLES USED: **deltoids**

This one is another favorite of mine. You really feel it in your obliques. If it starts to hurt your back, just drop to your knees and dip side to side.

1 Start in a plank position with your body raised on your forearms, making sure your elbows are directly underneath your shoulders.

2 Place your feet close together behind you, pushing your heels back. Keep your core engaged and your back, neck and shoulders in a straight line.

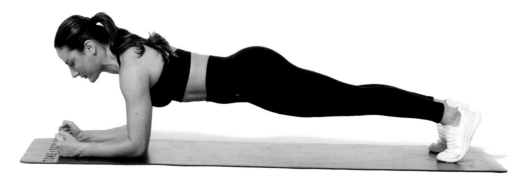

3 Rotate one hip down to the side, until you are hovering just above the floor.

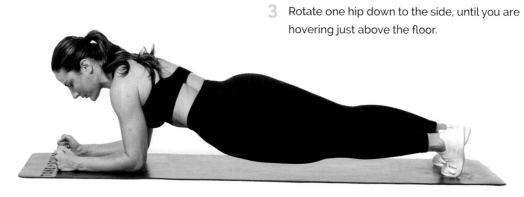

4 Return to the start position and repeat with the other hip.
Do 6–8 reps on each side.

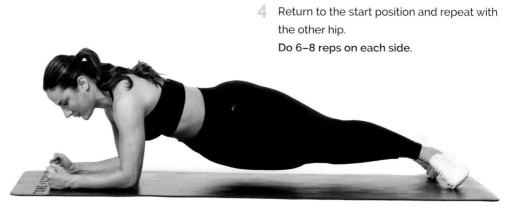

GROUP THREE:
UPPER BODY

BICYCLES

PRIMARY MUSCLES USED: **core**
SECONDARY MUSCLES USED: **obliques**

The bicycle is a traditional and very effective exercise that really engages your core muscles. Just be careful not to pull on your head and make sure your core doesn't dome. If your core domes (pops up) as you perform this exercise, it means it is not working as effectively as it could—go back to the start position and only come up as far as you can without your core doming.

1   Lie on your back on a mat with your hands behind your head, elbows out to the sides, knees bent up and feet lifted off the floor. Tilt your chin slightly, leaving about 4 inches of space between your chin and your chest—you should be able to see the tops of your knees.

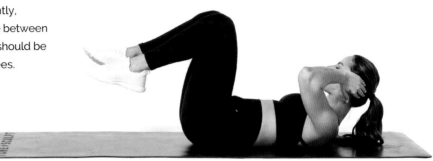

2   Gently pull your abdominal muscles inward, curl up and forward so that your head, neck and shoulder blades lift off the floor. Be mindful not to pull your head and neck up with your hands.

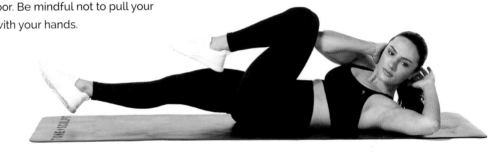

3   Straighten and lower your right leg until it hovers just above the floor. Crunch your abdominal muscles so that your right elbow aims to touch your left knee.

4   Pause for a couple of seconds before returning to the start position. Repeat on the other side. **Do 6–8 reps on each side.**

HEEL TOUCH

PRIMARY MUSCLES USED: **obliques**
SECONDARY MUSCLES USED: **core**

This is a simple move, but one that really works your obliques. I love it and always try to aim for my toes to achieve that added burn.

1   Lie on a mat on your back with your hands by your sides, knees bent up and feet planted on the floor hip distance apart. Raise your shoulders slightly off the floor.

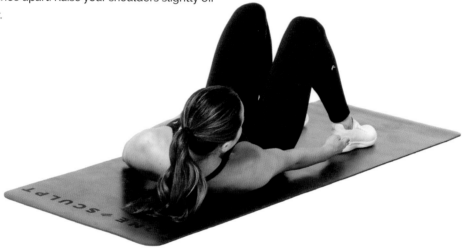

2   Reach for your heel with the hand on the same side, then bring the hand back and repeat on the opposite side, contracting your obliques each time.
Do 6–8 reps on each side.

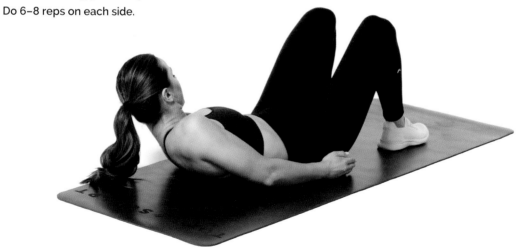

SIDE PLANK

PRIMARY MUSCLES USED: **core, obliques**
SECONDARY MUSCLES USED: **triceps, deltoids**

This is a tricky one but awesome for balance. The key is to make sure you don't let your hips or shoulders sink— you really need to push your forearm into the floor and your shoulder away from your neck. If you struggle with the full-body movement, do side plank on your knees. To progress this exercise, go onto your hand and do side plank crunches, bringing your knee in.

1   Lie on your side on a mat, leaning on your forearm, with your feet close together or stacked on top of each other. Make sure your forearm is directly below your shoulder.

2   Lift your hip off the floor so it forms a straight line with your shoulder and feet.

3   Hold for 30 seconds, then repeat on the other side.

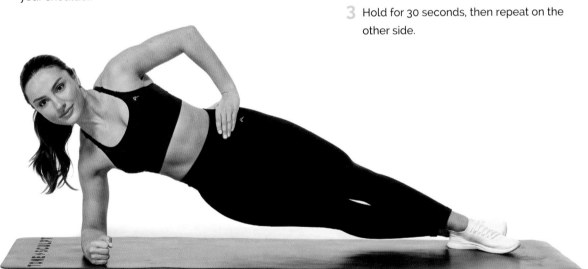

STRAIGHT-LEG TRICEP DIP

PRIMARY MUSCLES USED: **triceps**
SECONDARY MUSCLES USED: **core**

Tricep dips are among my favorites but also something I dread in my workouts. They completely isolate your triceps, and just by using your body weight you achieve so much through this simple movement. The challenge is to keep your elbows tucked in and try not to let your back move away from the chair or bench (whichever you choose to use). If it starts to hurt your back or you find it uncomfortable, bring your feet in and bend at the knees—work up to straight-leg tricep dips from here.

1 Start by placing the heels of your hands behind you on a bench or a chair. You will feel a slight stretch in your chest. Try to not let your elbows bow out—keep them in line with your shoulders.

2 Stretch your legs out in front and balance on your heels. Keep your back as close to the bench as possible (your back should stay in the same position throughout the movement).

3 Take a deep breath in and slowly lower your body, bending at the elbows until you are hovering off the floor—keep your back vertical at all times.

4 As you exhale, use your triceps to push yourself back up through the heels of your hands.
Do 12–15 reps.

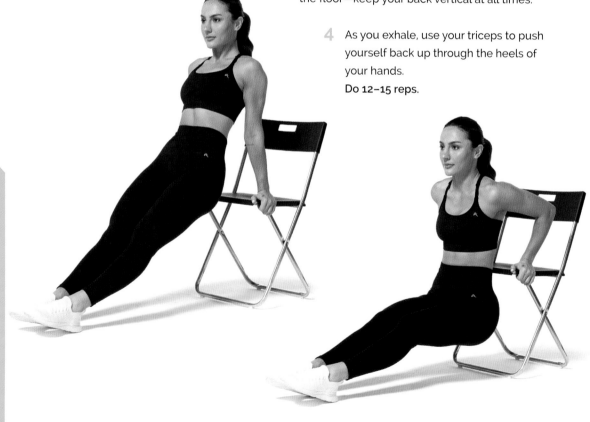

GROUP FOUR: UPPER BODY

STRAIGHT-LEG TRICEP DIP ON MAT

PRIMARY MUSCLES USED: **triceps**
SECONDARY MUSCLES USED: **core, glutes**

This is tough but a great move for your triceps and core—all you need is the floor and your body weight. To really challenge yourself, try to hover above the floor rather than resting on the mat with each tricep dip before returning to the starting position.

1 Sit on a mat with your hands behind you, legs straight in front of you, knees soft and in line with your toes.

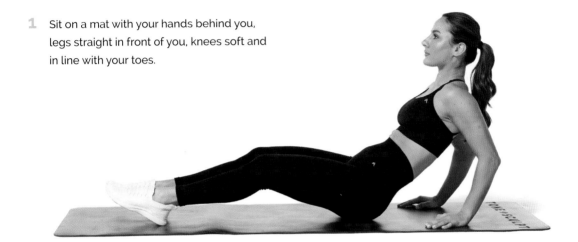

2 Lift your body weight up off the mat by pressing into the heels of your hands.

3 Keeping your legs straight, bend at the elbows as you use your triceps to lower your upper body down toward the floor.

4 Push up through the triceps to return to the starting position.
   Do 12–15 reps.

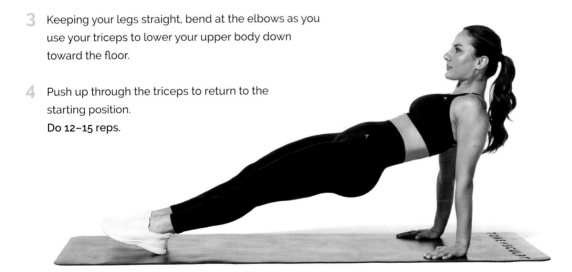

SEATED OVERHEAD TRICEP EXTENSION

PRIMARY MUSCLES USED: **triceps**

A seated overhead tricep extension is great if you experience back pain and want to add a little bit of extra resistance to fire up those triceps. You can also perform skull crushers, by lying down on a bench or mat and taking the dumbbell over your head to work your triceps. If you don't have a dumbbell, a water bottle or can of tomatoes can work instead—anything that can provide some resistance.

1 Sit down and hold a dumbbell in a vertical position, wrapping your palms around the handle at the top end.

2 Lift the dumbbell up over your head, keeping your elbows in. Keep your arms fully extended.

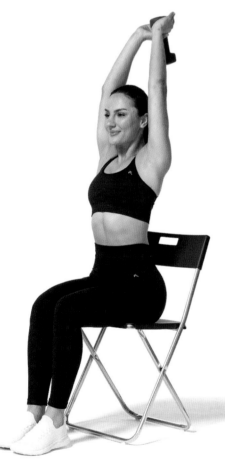

3 Using your forearms only, lower the dumbbell between your shoulders until you feel a stretch down your triceps, keeping your elbows still.

4 Extend back up and repeat the movement.
Do 12–15 reps.

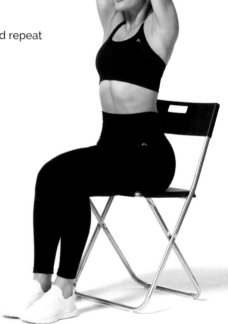

NARROW-INCLINE PUSH-UP

PRIMARY MUSCLES USED: triceps
SECONDARY MUSCLES USED: chest, trapezius, core

This is a great movement to fire up your chest and back muscles, as well as support your push-up progression. The key is to maintain that straight-line posture; don't let your hips sink down—it's really important to keep your core engaged throughout this movement.

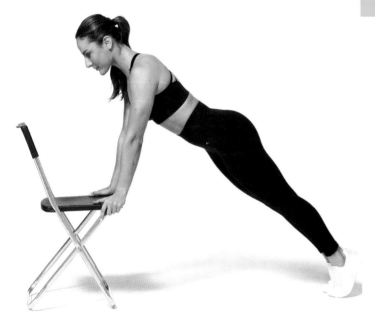

1   Begin by placing your hands on a bench or chair in front of you, shoulder width apart.

2   Stretch your legs out behind you, keeping your feet about hip distance apart, core engaged and back in line with your neck and shoulders. You should be on the balls of your feet with your heels pushed back.

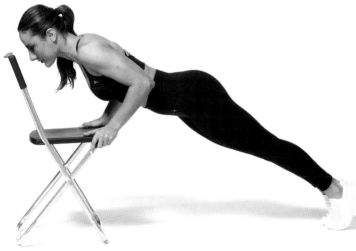

3   Maintaining a straight line throughout the movement, inhale and keep your elbows in as you lower your chest toward the bench.

4   Exhale as you push back into the start position.
Do 12–15 reps.

COCOON

PRIMARY MUSCLES USED: **core**

My favorite abs exercise, the cocoon works your entire core, and you can vary it to suit your level—you don't need to extend your legs all the way out, just go as far as you can. Try not to lift your head off the floor as this can strain it. To help you, you can start by just extending your legs in and out before introducing your arms into the movement. If your core domes (lifts up), you're going too far and need to work toward this extension—you want your core to stay as flat as possible throughout the movement.

1   Begin by lying on your back on a mat. Your legs should be straight and your arms extended behind your head.

2   Exhale as you engage your core and lift your legs, rotating your pelvis up, which will plant your lower back firmly on the floor. Your glutes will lift a little too.

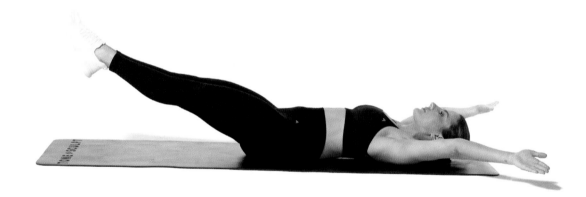

3   Lift your knees to your chest. As they come in, bring your hands round from behind you to touch your knees as you crunch in.

4   Pause for a few seconds and then extend your arms and legs out again (hovering off the floor) in the starting position.
Do 12–15 reps.

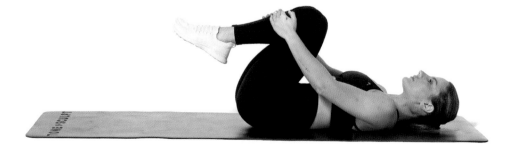

LEG RAISE

PRIMARY MUSCLES USED: **core**
SECONDARY MUSCLES USED: **quads**

This is a great move for your lower abdominal muscles. For a little extra support, place your fingers (not your whole hand) underneath your glutes. You can do alternating leg raises to begin with, or start in a tabletop position (knees bent at 90 degrees). To test yourself, lower your legs really slowly and bring them back up at the same pace.

1   Begin by lying on your back on a mat. Your legs should be straight and arms by your sides.

2   Exhale as you engage your core and lift your legs up straight above you.

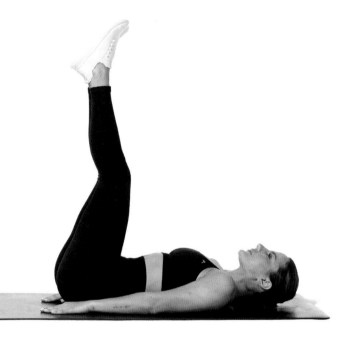

3   Slowly lower both legs down to a point where you feel a stretch in your core (make sure your core doesn't dome).

4   Hold for a few seconds before lifting your legs back up into the air.
    Do 12–15 reps.

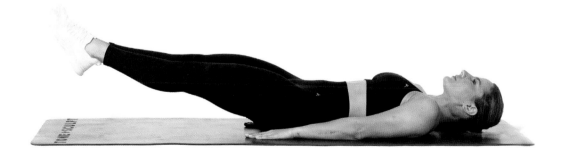

V-UP

PRIMARY MUSCLES USED: **core**
SECONDARY MUSCLES USED: **quads**

This one burns! It really challenges your balance and works your entire core. If you find you struggle to hold the V-up in the air, simply place your feet on the floor, keep your knees bent and perform a sit-up, reaching for the sky.

1 Begin by lying on your back on a mat with your arms by your sides and legs straight.

2 Lift your arms and legs so they are at a 45-degree angle in the air, keeping them straight.

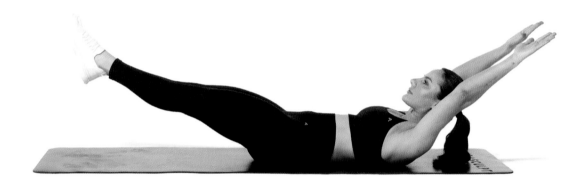

3 Continue to lift your legs and arms and lift up your body with your core, reaching for your toes. Pause and then return slowly to the floor.
Do **12–15 reps**.

SUPERMAN

PRIMARY MUSCLES USED: **glutes, chest**
SECONDARY MUSCLES USED: **rear deltoids, trapezius, lats**

These are great for strengthening and conditioning your back, glute and core muscles. You'll really feel a nice burn in your back and glutes—but it shouldn't feel painful, so try to avoid arching and lifting beyond what you can.

1 Begin by lying on the floor, facedown, with your arms reaching forward above your head. You may want to use a towel or something soft for your forehead to rest on.

2 Extend your legs straight out behind you.

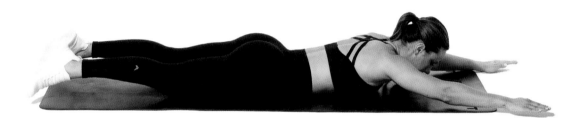

3 Keeping your core engaged, lift your head, shoulders and legs as far as you can off the floor without causing pain.

4 Pause and contract all your back muscles before returning to the floor.
Do 12–15 reps.

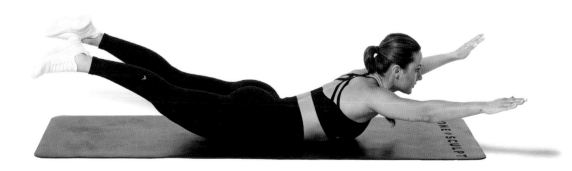

CLAM

PRIMARY MUSCLES USED: **glutes**
SECONDARY MUSCLES USED: **obliques**

Clams burn those glutes! This is such a great no-equipment exercise—it is super effective in engaging and firing up your glutes at the same time as engaging your obliques. By keeping your head, neck and shoulders in line, you are working the tops of your shoulders too. Positioning and form are key in this exercise as you are working hard to engage the glutes—always check your form before you begin.

1   Lie on a mat on your side with hips and shoulders in a straight line. Bend your knees, keeping the bottoms of your feet in line with your glutes.

2   Lift your body so your weight is on your lower elbow, directly under your shoulder. Place the other hand on your hip, or on the floor just in front of your chest for extra stability.

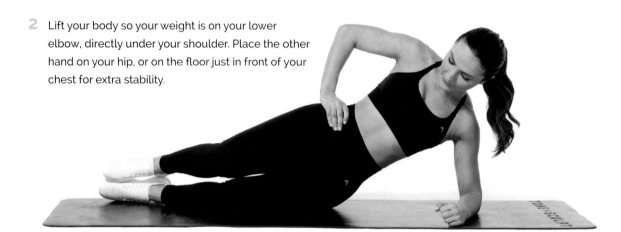

3   Your feet should be directly on top of one another and your hips neatly stacked.

4   Keeping your feet together, inhale and lift your top knee, opening up your legs as far as you can go without disturbing your hip alignment.

5   Exhale and bring your knee back to the starting position. Do all repetitions on one side before moving to the other side. **Do 12–15 reps on each side.**

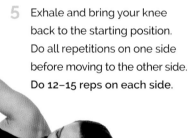

GROUP SIX:
LOWER BODY

FIRE HYDRANT

PRIMARY MUSCLES USED: **glutes**
SECONDARY MUSCLES USED: **core**

Fire hydrants are really effective no-equipment glute exercises. Not only do they fire up your glutes, but you are forced to keep your core engaged too—this is ideal for anyone with a sore back as it helps stabilize and strengthen the lower back. Try not to let your shoulder blades sink toward the floor or your back arch—imagine you are trying to balance a tray on your back and do your best to keep it in a tabletop position.

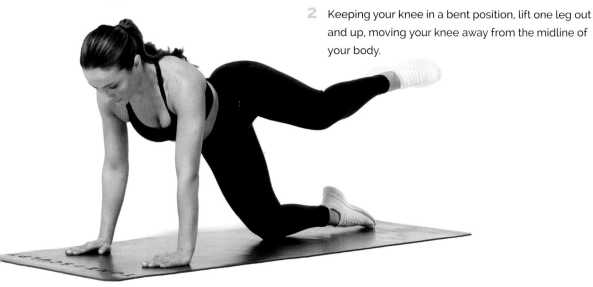

1 Position yourself on your hands and knees, with hands directly under your shoulders and knees directly under your hips.

2 Keeping your knee in a bent position, lift one leg out and up, moving your knee away from the midline of your body.

3 Lift your knee as far as you can without letting your lower back arch or bend, then pause at the top of the motion and return to the floor. If you can, let your knee hover above the floor rather than touching down before you repeat the movement. Do all repetitions on one side before moving to the other side.
Do 12–15 reps on each side.

DEADLIFT

PRIMARY MUSCLES USED: **hamstrings**
SECONDARY MUSCLES USED: **glutes**

1   Stand up straight with your feet shoulder
width apart. Grab a barbell or two dumbbells
in an overhand grip. Bend your knees slightly
and keep them stationary throughout the
exercise with your weight in your heels.

This is one of my favorite lower-body exercises.
As you get stronger and more confident, there are
so many variations of the deadlift you can try. It is
important to keep your core engaged throughout
the movement and your back completely straight
to prevent injury—form is really important with a
deadlift, so take your time with it and always ask
for help or correct your form if you experience
any back pain. If you do suffer from a bad back,
try sticking to fire hydrants or kickbacks until you
feel stronger.

2   Start lowering the barbell or dumbbells toward the midline
of your feet (your shoelaces), keeping your back completely
straight. You are hinging at the hips and pushing your glutes
back to get into the deadlift position.

3   Using just your hips as a hinge, return back to the
start position.
Do 12–15 reps.

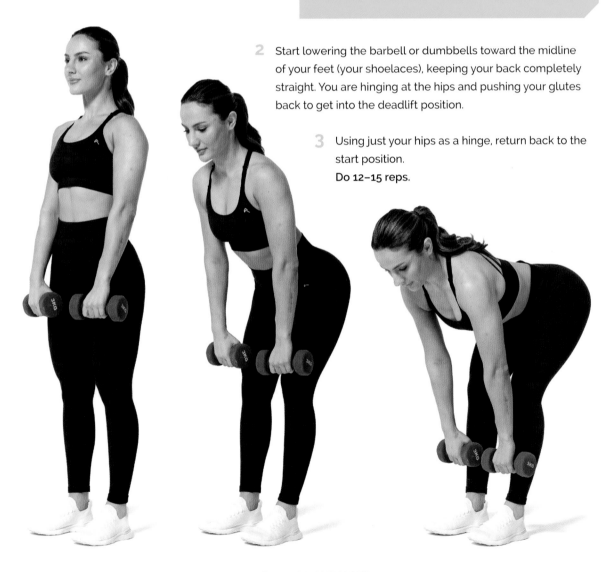

KICKBACK

PRIMARY MUSCLES USED: glutes
SECONDARY MUSCLES USED: core

Try your best to stop your hips from sinking or shoulders from hunching throughout this move—imagine you are balancing a tray on your back at all times.

1 Position yourself on your hands and knees, with hands directly under your shoulders and knees directly under your hips. Keep your back straight and core engaged at all times.

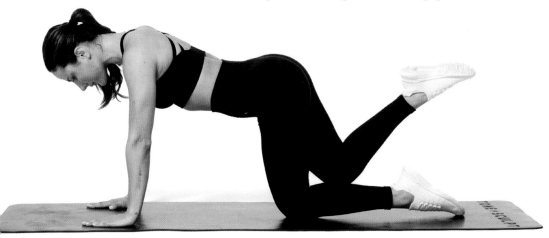

2 Keeping your hips still, lift one foot toward the ceiling, as if you are kicking up high with the back of your foot, leading with your heel. You should feel a contraction in your glutes.

3 Lift as far as you can without arching your lower back. Pause at the top, then lower your leg. If you can, let your knee hover above the floor rather than touching down before you repeat the motion. Do all repetitions on one side before moving on to the other leg. **Do 15–20 reps on each side.**

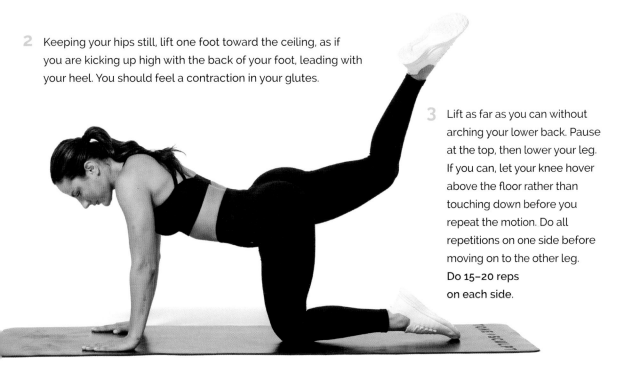

BODY-WEIGHT SQUAT

PRIMARY MUSCLES USED: **quads, glutes**
SECONDARY MUSCLES USED: **hamstrings**

The squat is an excellent lower-body compound movement and is super effective for strength and stamina. You can hold a dumbbell for an extra challenge or pulse up and down a few times as you sit into the squat. Hold the squat for a few seconds to engage your glutes and then squeeze them when you return to the standing position—the squeeze will help ease pressure on your back.

1   Stand with your feet just over hip distance apart, toes facing slightly outward, knees soft and in line with your toes.

2   Cross your hands over your chest and place them on your shoulders, keeping your elbows in line with your shoulders.

3   Brace your core, keeping it pulled in and engaged at all times throughout the movement. You should still be able to breathe throughout the movement.

4   Take a deep breath, push your hips back as if you are about to sit on a chair and sink your glutes down as far back as you can. Keep your knees in line with your toes and don't let them fall in. Keep your weight in your heels and make sure your back and chest are upright.

5   Pause for a few seconds at the bottom and, as you exhale, drive up through your heels and return to a standing position. Squeeze your glutes at the top. Do 12–15 reps.

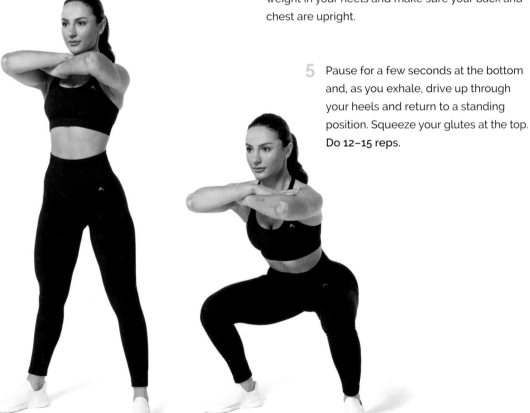

GROUP SEVEN: LOWER BODY

SUMO GOBLET SQUAT

PRIMARY MUSCLES USED: **glutes, quads**
SECONDARY MUSCLES USED: **hamstrings**

1 Hold a dumbbell at chest height, like you are holding a goblet or cup.

2 Stand with your feet wide apart (about double hip distance), toes at a 45-degree angle, knees soft and in line with your toes.

3 Brace your core, keeping it pulled in and engaged at all times throughout the movement. You should still be able to breathe throughout the movement.

Don't be fooled by a sumo squat—it makes your glutes and inner thighs burn! Sumo squats are great for really sculpting your peach. But don't feel like you have to do the splits to be in a sumo position. Your legs should be wide enough for you to feel your glutes and inner thighs contracting, but not so wide that you find it tricky to squat without your knees sinking in or your back beginning to hurt. If this happens, bring your legs in a little, or try it without a dumbbell to begin with. If you don't have a dumbbell, use a water bottle, a can of tomatoes—anything to add a little bit of resistance.

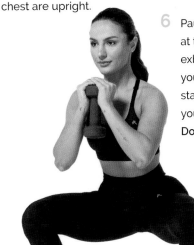

4 Take a deep breath, push your hips back as if you are about to sit on a chair and sink your glutes down as far back as you can.

5 Keep your knees in line with your toes and don't let them fall in. Keep your weight in your heels and make sure your back and chest are upright.

6 Pause for a few seconds at the bottom and, as you exhale, drive up through your heels and return to a standing position. Squeeze your glutes at the top. Do 12–15 reps.

SQUAT INTO CROSSOVER TOE TOUCH

PRIMARY MUSCLES USED: **quads, glutes**
SECONDARY MUSCLES USED: **hamstrings, core, obliques**

1   Stand with your feet just over hip distance apart, toes facing slightly outward, knees soft and in line with your toes. Place your hands at the sides of your head.

2   Brace your core, keeping it pulled in and engaged at all times throughout the movement. You should still be able to breathe throughout the movement.

3   Take a deep breath, push your hips back as if you are about to sit on a chair and sink your glutes down as far back as you can.

Crossover toe touches get your heart pumping while working your core and legs. I love this move—the added toe touch not only works your obliques but also fires up your hamstrings. If you want to take it up a notch, you can do a squat jump with a toe touch. Or if you want to work up to it, try touching your knee with your opposite elbow instead.

4   Keep your knees in line with your toes and don't let them fall in. Keep your weight in your heels and make sure your back and chest are upright. Pause for a few seconds.

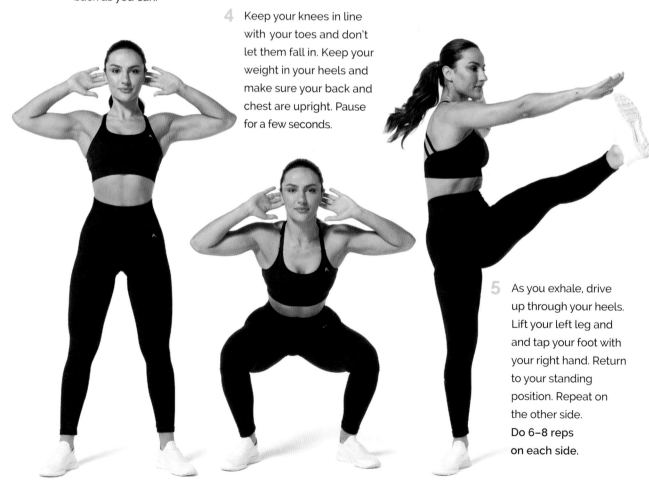

5   As you exhale, drive up through your heels. Lift your left leg and and tap your foot with your right hand. Return to your standing position. Repeat on the other side. **Do 6–8 reps on each side.**

NARROW-TO-WIDE SQUAT JUMPS

PRIMARY MUSCLES USED: **quads**
SECONDARY MUSCLES USED: **glutes, calves**

1 Stand with your feet just under hip width apart, feet facing forward and knees in line with your toes.

2 Take a deep breath in and start by doing a regular squat—push your hips back as if you are about to sit on a chair.

3 Keeping your core engaged, exhale and jump up explosively.

These jumps will burn. Trust me when I say they are a killer and an awesome addition to any workout. They add cardio and resistance, and they train all the muscles in your lower body. If you find the jumping in and out a little too much, perform standard jumping squats or try squatting from a standard to a narrow squat without the jump.

4 As you land, bring your feet further apart, just over shoulder width apart, and sink into a wide squat, keeping your knees in line with your toes.

5 Take another deep breath, jump up explosively and this time land back into the narrow squat you started with.
Do 12–15 reps.

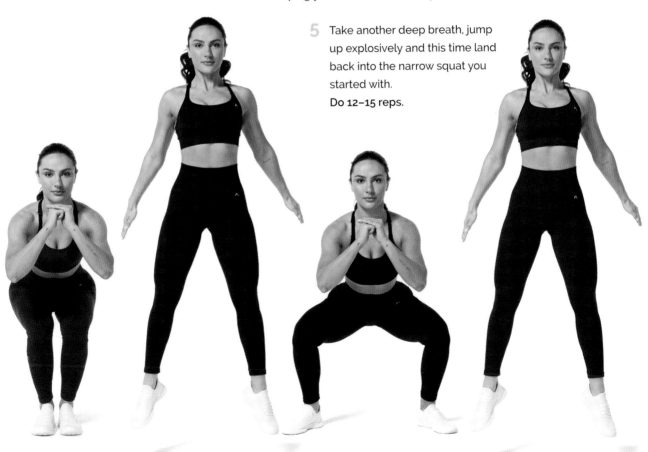

LUNGE WITH DUMBBELLS

PRIMARY MUSCLES USED: **quads**
SECONDARY MUSCLES USED: **glutes**

Lunges are great lower-body compound movements. As a unilateral (one-sided) movement, they are ideal for strengthening muscles on each side of the body in turn and helping you recognize and correct any imbalances too. If you find lunging forward hard on your knees, lunge backward instead—it eases the pressure a little.

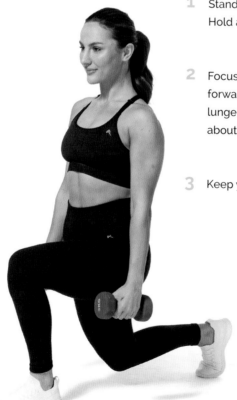

1   Stand up straight with your feet shoulder width apart. Hold a dumbbell in each hand.

2   Focus on a point in front of you as you take a big step forward, inhale and bend your back knee as you lunge into position. Both knees should be bent at about a 90-degree angle.

3   Keep your chest upright and try not to look down.

4   Return to your starting position and repeat on the other side.
    Do 6–8 reps on each side.

LUNGE PULSE

PRIMARY MUSCLES USED: **quads**
SECONDARY MUSCLES USED: **glutes**

Lunge pulses are an absolute burner and keep your muscles under tension throughout the duration of the exercise. Enjoy!

1   Start with your feet shoulder width apart and your hands on your hips.

2   Focus on a point in front of you as you take a big step forward. Inhale and bend your knees as you lunge into position. Both knees should be bent at about a 90-degree angle.

3   Keep your chest upright and try not to look down.

4   Pulse up and down by about 4 inches, then return to your starting position. Repeat on the other side. **Do 6–8 reps on each side.**

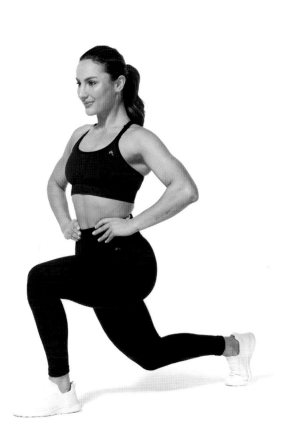
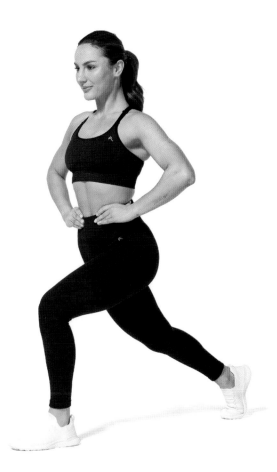

SPLIT SQUAT WITH DUMBBELLS

PRIMARY MUSCLES USED: quads, hamstrings
SECONDARY MUSCLES USED: glutes

1   Start by standing with your back to a bench or chair, holding a dumbbell in each hand. Keep the dumbbells on the outsides of your legs throughout this exercise so they are not in the way.

2   Place one foot on the chair behind you, with the other foot facing forward. Keep your knees in line with your toes and keep your core engaged throughout to help with balance.

Split squats are among my favorite exercises. They really challenge your balance while keeping your legs under tension throughout the movement—the burn feels amazing! It can take a while to get the split squat right as you need to check your position, making sure your legs are at the right distance from one another to allow you to squat back into position. Some people place the front of their back foot flat on the bench behind them (sole facing up); others place their toes down on the bench with sole facing down. It really depends on flexion in your ankle and what feels comfortable. So play around and see what works for you—you can try it without dumbbells to begin too.

3   Your upper body will be at a slight angle, bending forward to allow you to complete the range of movement.

4   Lower your body as if squatting back by bending the front knee—you will need to make sure there is enough space between your legs to allow you to sink into the position.

5   Drive back up through your heel to your standing position. Do all repetitions on one side before moving on to the other leg. **Do 6–8 reps on each side.**

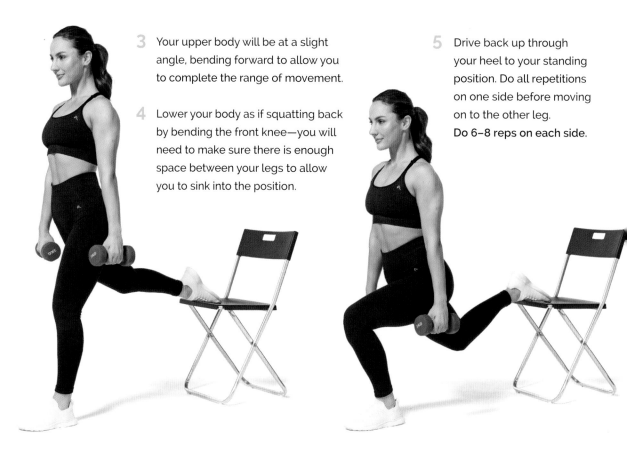

LUNGE JUMPS

PRIMARY MUSCLES USED: quads, glutes
SECONDARY MUSCLES USED: hamstrings

Lunge jumps bring a bit of fun to workouts. All I'll say is breathe and grit your teeth through them...you will learn to love them, I promise! If you find the jumping hurts your back or is a little too much for your knees, stick to body-weight lunges.

1 Start with your feet shoulder width apart. Hold your arms straight out in front of you with hands held together.

2 Place one foot behind you as if you are lunging back, both knees at a 90-degree angle.

3 Take a deep breath in and, as you exhale, jump up explosively and swap your legs around so that when you land you are lunging back on the other leg. Repeat on the other side.
Do 6–8 reps on each side.

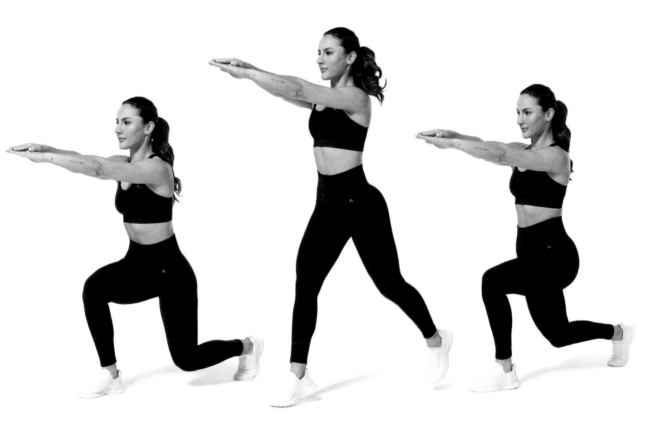

GLUTE BRIDGE

PRIMARY MUSCLES USED: **glutes**
SECONDARY MUSCLES USED: **core**

Glute bridges are a great exercise, not only for muscle strength, but for posture, balance and back pain too. The trick is to keep your core engaged at all times and make sure you are driving through your heels and lifting your hips up high. Add a dumbbell to your hips or a resistance band just above your knees for an added challenge.

1 Lie faceup on a mat, knees bent and feet flat on the floor. Keep your knees in line with your toes at all times, arms next to you.

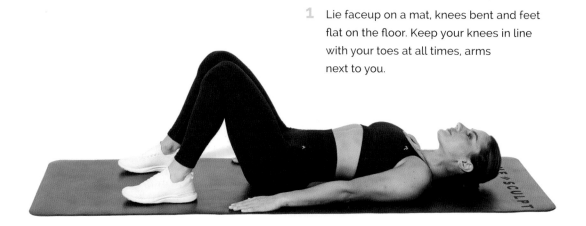

2 Keep your core engaged and exhale. Pushing through your heels, lift your hips off the floor and into the air until your knees, hips and shoulders form a straight line.

3 Squeeze your glutes and hold for a few seconds before returning to the floor. **Do 12–15 reps.**

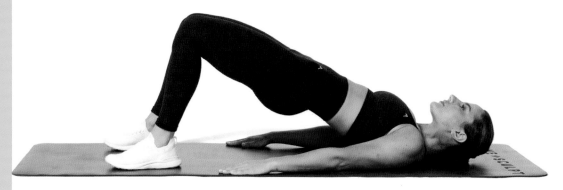

HIP THRUST

PRIMARY MUSCLES USED: **glutes**
SECONDARY MUSCLES USED: **hamstrings, core**

This is my favorite glute exercise. If doing this exercise at the gym, you can use a barbell. Just make sure your setup is safe and secure—seek assistance from a personal trainer or gym instructor.

1   Start by sitting on the floor with your back against a chair or bench, knees bent and feet flat on the floor.

2   Grab a dumbbell and place it across your hips. This will be your start position.

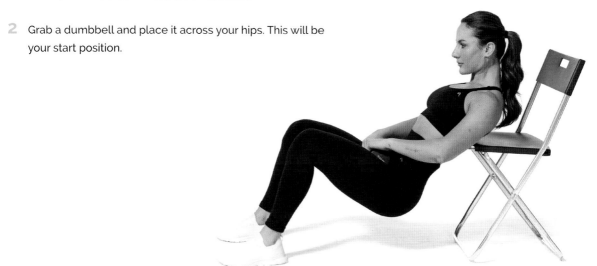

3   Driving through your heels and looking forward (not up), thrust your hips up, raising the dumbbell until your body almost looks like a tabletop. Your back (just by your bra strap) should stay against the bench at all times.

4   Hold for a few seconds and squeeze your glutes before returning to the start position.
    Do 10–15 reps.

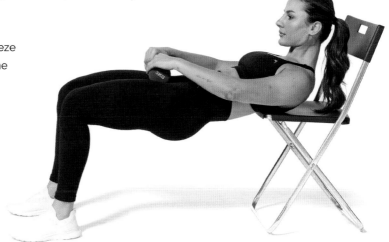

DUMBBELL LATERAL LUNGE & RAISE

PRIMARY MUSCLES USED: quads, side delts
SECONDARY MUSCLES USED: glutes

This is a challenging full-body movement, great for resistance and stamina. It really challenges your balance and core strength too. If you find you do not feel much in your glutes as you lunge from side to side, simply widen your stance. If you find it starts to hurt your back, try using lighter weights for the lateral raises.

1   Stand up straight with your feet hip width apart. Hold a dumbbell in each hand. Feet should be at a slight angle turning outward.

2   Step out wide to the side, bend one knee and lunge, sitting back to keep your knee in line with your toes. Your other leg should be straight and stretched out.

3   When in the lunge position, keep your chest upright and core engaged. Lift each dumbbell laterally to each side, keeping a slight bend in your elbows.

4   Return your arms to the middle and repeat on the other side. **Do 6–8 reps on each side.**

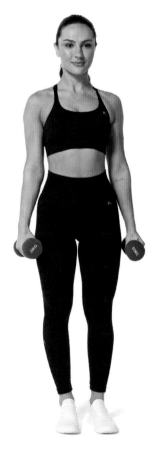
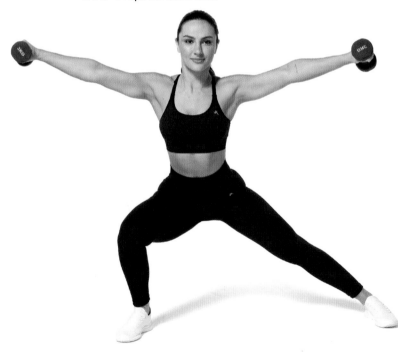

GLUTE BRIDGE WALK

PRIMARY MUSCLES USED: **glutes, hamstrings**
SECONDARY MUSCLES USED: **core, quads**

Glute bridge walks are great for your hamstrings. So versatile, they don't need any equipment and make a great addition to any lower-body workout.

1   Lie faceup on a mat, knees bent and feet flat on the floor. Keep your knees in line with your toes at all times, arms next to you with palms facing down.

2   Keep your core engaged and exhale. Pushing through your heels, lift your hips off the floor and into the air until your knees, hips and shoulders form a straight line. Lift one leg to slightly more than a 90-degree angle.

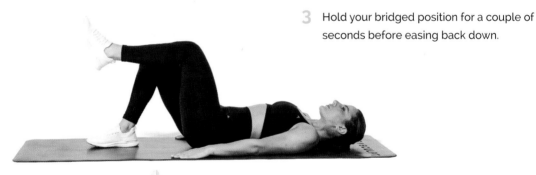

3   Hold your bridged position for a couple of seconds before easing back down.

4   Repeat on the other side in one smooth motion, as though you are walking on air. **Do 10–12 reps on each side.**

STEP-UP

PRIMARY MUSCLES USED: quads, glutes
SECONDARY MUSCLES USED: hamstrings

Step-ups are great, dynamic moves that really challenge your lower-body muscles using little equipment. As with most body-weight movements, you can get creative with this one by adding a knee crunch at the end (where you drive the knee up to contract your abdominal muscles) or a glute kickback (where you kick your heel back at the top of the movement to feel a squeeze in your glutes).

1 Stand in front of a bench, chair or raised platform, at a height that you can step up onto without causing discomfort.

2 Step up with one foot.

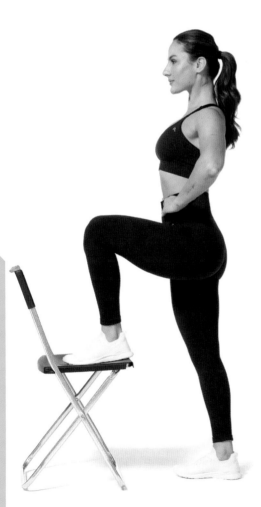

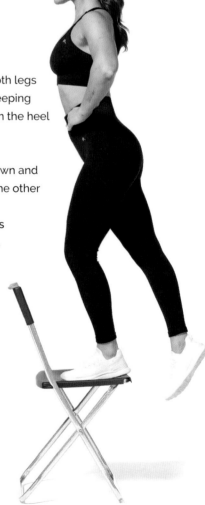

3 Straighten both legs and lift up, keeping your weight in the heel of your foot.

4 Step back down and repeat with the other foot.
   Do 12–15 reps on each side.

GROUP TEN: LOWER BODY

REVERSE LUNGE WITH LEG LIFT

PRIMARY MUSCLES USED: **glutes, quads**
SECONDARY MUSCLES USED: **core, hamstrings**

This body-weight movement really challenges your glutes and fires up your core too. For an extra challenge, you can hold a dumbbell for a bit more resistance.

1 Stand with your hands on your hips with feet hip distance apart.

2 Lift one foot and lunge back, taking your foot behind you, keeping on the balls of your feet and ensuring both knees are at a 90-degree angle.

3 Bring your foot back in to stand up straight, but continue the movement forward, lifting your leg in front of you.

4 Return to the starting position. Do all repetitions on one side before moving to the other side.
Do 6–8 reps on each side.

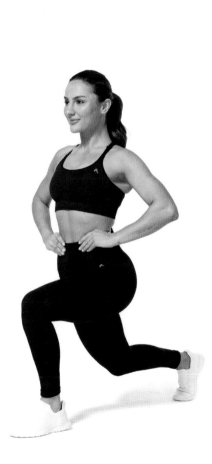
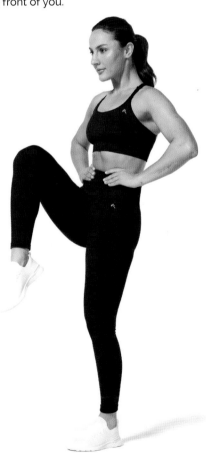

DUMBBELL CURTSEY LUNGE

PRIMARY MUSCLES USED: **quads, glutes**
SECONDARY MUSCLES USED: **hamstrings**

The curtsey lunge is a firm favorite and a really nice way to change up a traditional lunge. It targets your glutes and inner thighs. You may need to rotate your front foot in slightly, depending on your flexion.

1   Stand with your feet shoulder width apart, holding a dumbbell in each hand by your hips.

2   Place your right foot a little behind your left foot.

3   Take a big step back and to the side, as if about to curtsey. Lunge down, keeping your chest upright and feet in line with your toes.

4   Return to the starting position and repeat on the other side.
    Do 6–8 reps on each side.

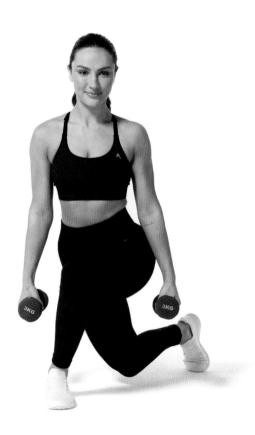

STANDING LEG ABDUCTION INTO STRAIGHT-LEG KICKBACK

PRIMARY MUSCLES USED: **glutes**
SECONDARY MUSCLES USED: **core**

This is a great movement to really wake up your glute muscles and can be done as part of a warm-up or your main workout. It looks easy, but it really burns. It's so great, you can even do it while you're cooking or waiting for the kettle to boil! As it is a unilateral movement, it's great for strengthening your glute muscles on each side, while helping with balance too. You can hold on to something to begin with to help you balance.

1 Stand up nice and tall and place your hands on your hips. Keep your core engaged at all times and try not to arch your back.

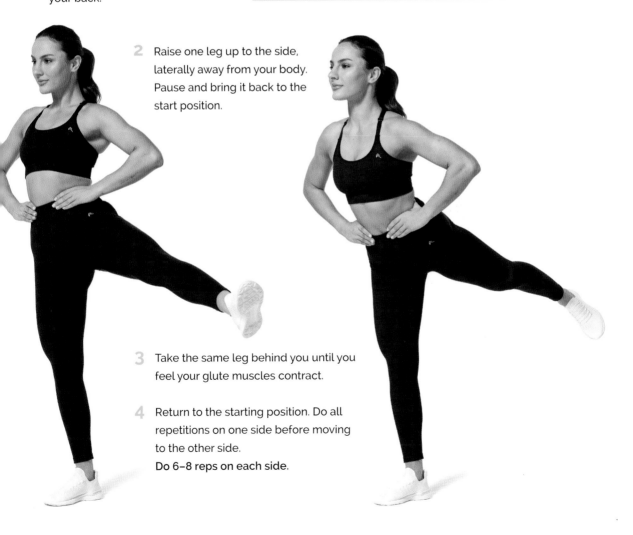

2 Raise one leg up to the side, laterally away from your body. Pause and bring it back to the start position.

3 Take the same leg behind you until you feel your glute muscles contract.

4 Return to the starting position. Do all repetitions on one side before moving to the other side.
Do 6–8 reps on each side.

BURPEE

PRIMARY MUSCLES USED: **quads, core**
SECONDARY MUSCLES USED: **chest, calves**

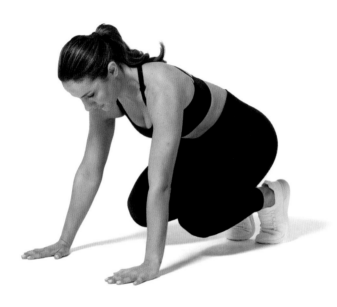

1   Start by standing up straight, feet hip distance apart.

2   Crouch down and place your hands on the floor.

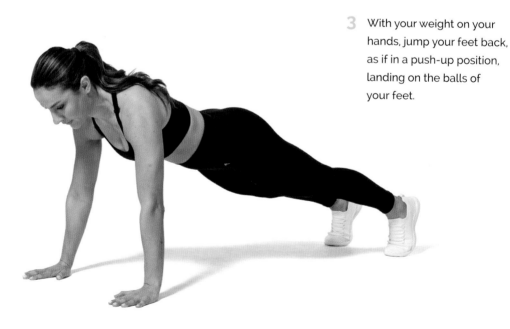

3   With your weight on your hands, jump your feet back, as if in a push-up position, landing on the balls of your feet.

Burpees are a real military-style movement, great for stamina and strength combined. As you progress, you can have a lot of fun with this exercise by incorporating a press-up or mountain climber too.

4 Keep your core engaged and jump your feet back in, then jump up explosively to the starting position.
Do 10–12 reps.

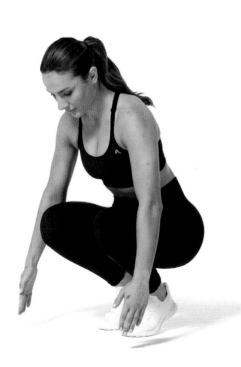

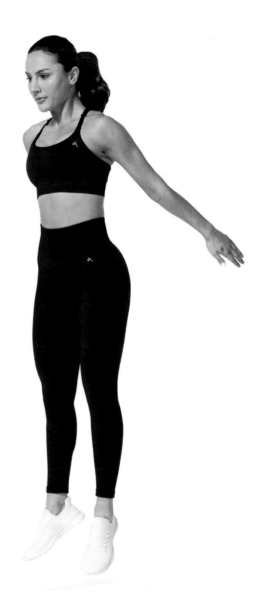

PLANK WALK IN & OUT

PRIMARY MUSCLES USED: **core**
SECONDARY MUSCLES USED: **chest, quads**

1 Stand up straight. Soften your
knees and then bend at the waist
to touch the floor.

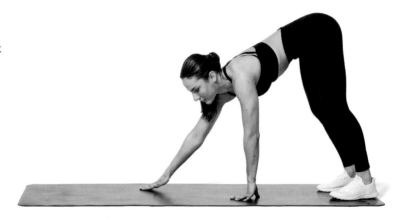

2 With your weight on the balls
of your feet, crawl forward on
your hands into a high plank.

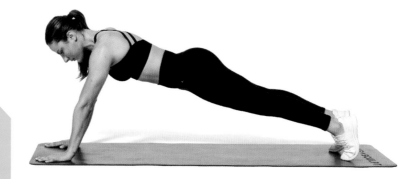

This move looks simple, but
those crawl-ins and -outs
really challenge your core,
legs and stamina. For an added
challenge, why not stand up
in between each movement
or add in an upright row? To
perform an upright row, grab
a kettlebell, dumbbell or water
bottle and hold it in between
your hands, arms straight down
in front of you. Pull the weight
up toward your chin so your
elbows point outward and
upward, forming a triangle with
your elbows and chin.

3 With your core nice and
tight, crawl back to your
start position.
Do 10–12 reps.

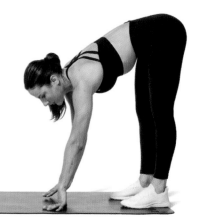

PLANK JACK

PRIMARY MUSCLES USED: **core**
SECONDARY MUSCLES USED: **triceps, glutes**

Plank jacks are a great way to challenge your plank progression and get your heart racing. If you're not keen on jumping in and out, don't worry—just step in and out with one foot at a time.

1 Start in a plank position with your elbows directly under your shoulders, feet close together behind you and your back in line with your head, neck and shoulders.

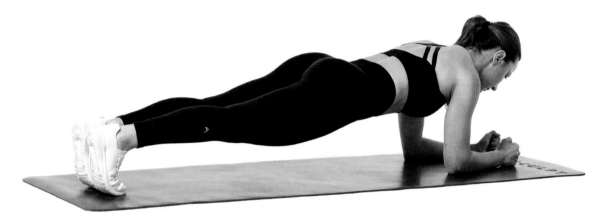

2 Keeping your core tight, jump out with both feet as if forming an upside-down V. Take a breath and jump your feet back in.
   Do 10–15 reps.

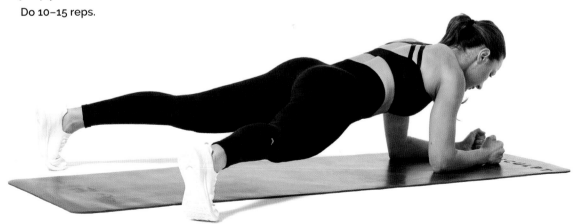

KNEELING SQUAT
INTO SQUAT JUMP

PRIMARY MUSCLES USED: **quads**
SECONDARY MUSCLES USED: **glutes, calves**

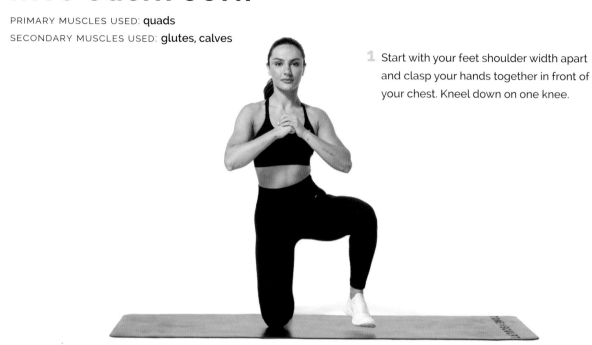

1 Start with your feet shoulder width apart and clasp your hands together in front of your chest. Kneel down on one knee.

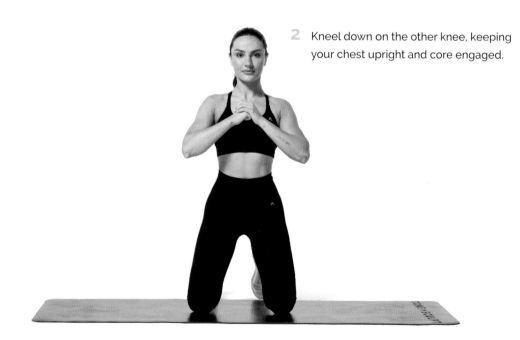

2 Kneel down on the other knee, keeping your chest upright and core engaged.

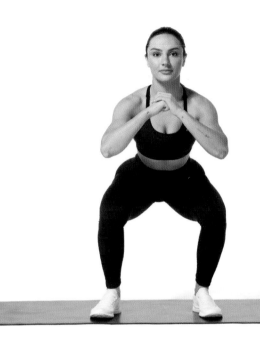

This is a real quad and glute burner. I love adding this to my workouts as it really challenges my strength and stamina.

3 Step back up into a squat position.

4 Jump up explosively, landing back into the start position.
Do 10–15 reps.

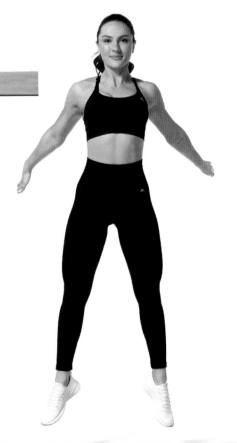

YOUR JOURNEY STARTS HERE

I've written this book with ease and fun in mind. I want you to remember that taking care of your fitness and health can be a habit that you enjoy and do without question. The workouts and recipes are all a part of my everyday life, and they can be a part of yours too.

You might be pleasantly surprised by the range of recipes in this book, now that you've read through them. Remember, food is your friend, not your enemy—as clichéd as that might sound! It's all about finding a balance that works for you and enjoying the process at the same time. Eat a balanced plate and wholesome foods, but enjoy that pizza every now and again too.

The best thing about learning to cook these recipes is that you will become more and more familiar with the ingredients. When you're out and about or on vacation at a restaurant, you don't need to feel anxious about the menu or worry about "indulging" either. Your knowledge of food and cooking will naturally increase, and you'll be able to recognize the different ingredients and balanced dishes without feeling you're missing out on tasty options. Whatever you do, remember you don't need to punish yourself. When you learn to cook these recipes and work with different ingredients, you'll feel more and more confident with your food choices—and you'll fall in love with food too!

The human body is an incredible machine. It is not your enemy but your greatest weapon—and I truly mean that. The workouts in this book are a good start but are great for longevity too. If you want to go further with them, progress with heavier weights, take it to the gym or extend the duration of your workout. As you get more confident with form and technique, you'll notice that you want to train more and more—it's such a positive feeling. Always remember, the daily walk, those 20-minute workouts and even the one burpee a day you've committed to will become a habitual part of your routine well into your seventies. You'll be running around with your grandchildren, reaching the highest shelves in your house and dancing around feeling ageless! If there is any goal to truly aim for, it's that one—to live a long, happy and healthy life feeling your best, every single day.

Everyone's fitness journey is unique; everyone's food preferences are different. Now that you've come to the end of the book, I don't want you just to close it and put it on a shelf. I want you to implement it into your lifestyle. Bookmark the recipes that work for you and add the ingredients to your shopping list. Write down the exercises you like the look of and use the guided formats (see pages 184–190) to design your workout. Keep in mind, life is not perfect, and it's not meant to be either—we all have ups and downs, and there will be days when even with the best will in the world, your workout just doesn't have a place. That's OK. There are so many different ways to move, to feel well, and there is always tomorrow. Reset, refocus and remember YOU matter!

Thank you so much for trusting me as your trainer. Your well-being needs are unique, and I hope this book has given you the tools to put your fitness and health first. There is no rush, no competition—you're doing this for you and only you.

And remember, you're part of the familia now. There is a whole community alongside you, eager to cheer you on to becoming the very best version of yourself!

INDEX

ACKNOWLEDGMENTS

I am so thankful and grateful for the opportunity to share the book I wish I had when I started focusing on my fitness and routine.

I can't thank the team at Octopus enough for trusting me to write this for you. This book would not be possible without Natalie, Jenny, Yasia, Ella, Megan and an entire team that believes in my ethos. Thank you so much.

Zahara, thank you for bringing this book to life.

Fitness and nutrition are habits, and our habits come from discipline, consistency and long-term thinking. For that, I have to thank my wonderful mum. Despite the difficulties we faced growing up, from moving countries to working around the clock, my mum always made sure there was a wholesome, balanced and nutritious meal on the table every night.

She taught me that food is so much more than fuel—it is a lifestyle and one that can bring a family together, feed your soul and make you happy. She taught me to cook, to enjoy the process and eat everything! I honestly believe it was this approach that helped me with my fitness, discipline and habits too. She taught me that anything can be achieved, so long as you believe in yourself and stay focused, humble and consistent.

Thank you, Mum—this book is for you.

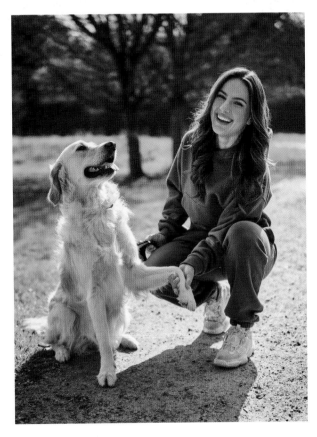

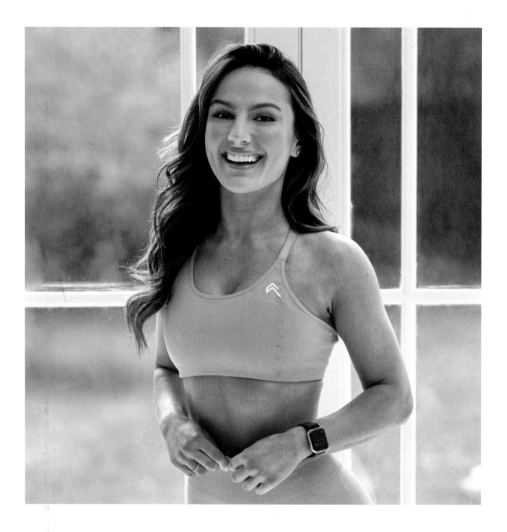

Krissy Cela first turned to fitness during a particularly challenging time in her life and started posting her workouts on social media while studying for a law degree. Her following quickly grew, and she now has a loyal and devoted community of more than 3.5 million followers on Instagram, Facebook and YouTube who she lovingly refers to as her "familia."

In January 2019 she launched the smash hit app, Tone & Sculpt, comprising more than five hundred workouts, a community forum and a meal planner fully customizable for each user's dietary needs. The app achieved more than 250,000 downloads in its first six months alone.

Krissy's first book, *Do This for You*, was published in January 2021.